10 INSPIRATIONAL FITNESS AND NUTRITION SHORT STORIES

How to overcome personal challenges with fitness and nutrition in the modern world

By Michael S. Parker

EBook:
ISBN-13: 978-1-7350614-1-2

Paperback:
ISBN-13: 978-1-7350614-0-5

Library of Congress Control Number:
2020908863

Cover by Turning Heads Designs

This book is dedicated to all my clients and those who struggle with fitness and nutrition but never give up.

Table of Contents

ABOUT THE AUTHOR

For nearly two decades, Michael S. Parker has worked as a fitness professional and executive-level manager. He has earned multiple credentials from the National Academy of Sports Medicine, National Exercise & Sports Trainers Association and the Spencer Institute. He is a Certified Master Personal Trainer, Lifestyle & Weight Management Coach and Functional Movement Specialist.

He also holds a business degree from the University of Phoenix. Michael is a former college instructor and consultant to the Advanced Personal Training and Exercise Science program offered by Bryan University. Further, he is an advisor, author and consultant to multiple fitness companies and publications in the United States.

In 2019 and 2020, Michael was ranked as one of the top online personal trainers and habit coaches in the world by Consumers Advocate. He is an avid outdoors person and spends much of his time backpacking, mountaineering, snowboarding, motorcycling and traveling.

Michael is the Founder and CEO of Forge Fitness and Nutrition Coaching. Forge provides highly custom online fitness and nutrition coaching services designed to accommodate all fitness levels. Forge works with individuals and corporations to improve habit-based wellness strategies in over 30 countries around the world and counting.

INTRODUCTION

In my coaching calls with clients, I find it remarkably useful to share stories about other clients and how they maintain their own motivation.

Because clients respond so well to the stories of others struggling but still working to overcome their own challenges, I compiled a few true short stories directly from my clients to share publicly to inspire others. It is my hope that some content in this book resonates with you and adds value.

Because I wanted to be sure the tone and personality of each client was unchanged, I did truly little editing on these stories. Grammar, punctuation, and typos were addressed, of course, but otherwise, these are not altered.

I kept my clients' writing styles and unique sentence phrasing untouched to make each story unique and true to form as possible. I was so pleased that a good number of my clients participated and submitted their personal tales.

I also wanted the book to be rather short, so we felt that having no more than ten stories over one thousand words but not over three thousand would make this a fun and easy read.

It was a tough selection process because I had over ten submitted and wanted to make sure there was a good variety of gender, age, location, and life circumstances. Yes, I had far more women contribute than men and felt that the stories that made it to publication had the best chances of inspiring.

Therefore, there are a few more female than male personal stories. As I was compiling and editing these stories, I noticed several trends. First, many titles were similar and concerned working on becoming the best you can be, despite the difficulties.

Second, many stories share points of pain and conditions that usually cause people to quit. Third, none of these fine people that shared their stories have given up and despite the challenges, continue to work on themselves daily. These are not necessarily success stories because wellbeing is a journey and the destination ends when we pass from this earth.

These stories are about people who have struggled, get frustrated, suffer injuries or distractions. What makes the stories inspiring is that despite these obstacles, each of these people work to adjust their attitude and never, ever give up.

Also, there were no requirements that I or Forge Fitness and Nutrition Coaching be recognized or plugged by a contributor. Any mention of myself or my company by a client is coincidental and not coerced.

But I admit, it was heartwarming to read some of the nice things mentioned. At the end of each story, I have included some of my own professional notes and coaching to add even more value.

THE COVID-19 PANDEMIC

I was inspired to collect and share these stories based on the unfortunate life-altering events of early 2020. There has been an incredible loss of livelihood, life, and security over the past few months and this has greatly affected motivation and focus of so many.

No doubt about it, we are experiencing some interesting and challenging times as a planet, country, and individuals because of COVID19.

Once the mandated isolations began, I noticed several regrettable trends both from coaching calls and looking at client program adherence. I would like to share three alarming observations about some general trends and give additional encouragement aside from the short stories in this book.

First, in coaching calls, many clients expressed major motivational issues to get their home workouts done after gyms closed. Ironically, those clients that already only workout form home were experiencing the same motivational issues as those who used to work out in gyms before the pandemic.

The quantity of missed workouts by my clients around the world escalated quickly. This has much to do with the major lifestyle shift we have all had to endure and the breaking of routine.

What compounds this issue is many people are finding they have more free time in isolation but struggle to use that time for productive activities.

On coaching calls with clients, I heard more about all the new video streaming shows than successful workout and nutrition management. Second, I got overwhelming reports about excessive snacking and loss of control on food management and even alcohol consumption for many clients increased.

Between meal plans being harder to follow because of store inventory and quarantines, folks reverted to boredom eating. Third, most of us are concerned about financial outlooks and potential long-term economic suffering.

I agree, this period of isolation, uncertainty and perhaps fear can cause a sort of paralysis. I have recognized a few changes in my own consistency with workouts, which I have addressed.

My message for each of you is one of hope, encouragement and understanding. Now more than ever, we must try to maximize our wellness. Fit bodies and determined minds are a force for wellbeing and by keeping up with your workouts and dialing nutrition we can make a positive shift considering the circumstances.

One client had said, "When this is all over, we get to choose what we pick back up." I found this to be an extraordinarily inspiring thought considering where we are as a community.

Every day, we get to decide what we do and how we will emerge from this pandemic. Every day accumulates and you get to decide, do you come out of this better or worse?

The good news is you have all the power to make that decision. Of course, we have conditions and external pressures that can change our normal routines, but we need to be agile.

Decide today to be the best you can despite the economy or pandemic. Stay home, internally focus on the wellness of yourself, your family and community.

Think of every new day as an opportunity to better yourself and take the time to focus energy towards positive outcomes. I also encourage you to connect with friends or family through technology and share your hope.

Instead of streaming ten hours of mindless TV about big cat cult leaders each day, video chat your loved ones who may be feeling lonely or isolated as well.

This is also an excellent time to strengthen relationships with those with whom you are sharing this isolation. Get your whole family in on bodyweight workouts or some yoga.

Now is not the time to quit; it is time to rally as a person, community, and nation. This will pass and you get to decide how you emerge. I wish you all health and joy, despite these troubling times and hope these short stories inspire you.

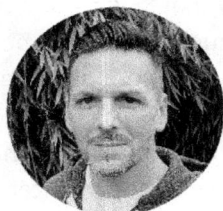

RYAN BATURA

"Washed Up, Has Been
Working to Stay in The Game"

I began riding and racing motorcycles & bicycles at age 5 under the tutelage of my father, a hardened veteran of professional flat track racing of the late 1950's. It was clarified almost immediately that toughness, physical fitness and strength were compulsory to be competitive. I found the rigorous training and riding to be both fun and rewarding.

At 24 years old, I had already amassed quite a laundry list of minor injuries and resulting orthopedic surgeries, but still felt largely unaffected by them. However, late in that season, I suffered a back injury while off-road racing that would prove to be life-changing. Initially, I thought I had just jarred my back and was unaware of any major problem. Then hardly able to lift my leg to dismount the motorcycle, my situation quickly became much more apparent.

In almost the same moment I noticed my right boot seemed to weigh about 100lbs, I felt a warm sensation in my right leg. Alas, in the ultimate moment of humility, I had lost control of my bladder and had relieved myself right then and there.

I remember so clearly that "Rich," one of the crew members who was always joking, laughing and in a perpetual state of yucking it up, went absolutely stone serious as he realized the type of trouble I was in.

Shortly after the arrival of the EMT's, things go a bit fuzzy. Things focused once again in recovery after an emergency Laminectomy surgery to relieve the compression on my spinal cord due to a ruptured L4 disc.

It was explained that a spinal fusion would be necessary as soon as possible to immobilize the damaged vertebrae. A good friend and fellow rider insisted that I receive a second opinion from a doctor who specializes in treating professional athletes.

A few weeks later, after receiving a thorough physical examination and reviewing my medical history, it was suggested that I forestall the spinal fusion surgery in exchange for an aggressive physical therapy program focusing on physiology, core strength and mobility.

The belief was that with my strong foundation in fitness and training, it was possible that I might achieve a higher level of recovery than if I had the spinal fusion done. The stakes had never been higher for dedicating myself to a training program.

These days it seems like my insurance requires me to changes doctors every few years, and each time I meet a new GPMD the reaction is similar upon reviewing my health history. With so many traumatic body injuries and surgical repairs/implants, the conversation is almost textbook in the talking points. Degenerative conditions, living with chronic pain, depression, drug therapy and so on.

It's ironic that during a time when consistent training is key to my health and mobility, my ability to do so is so rapidly diminishing due to all the post-traumatic pain, arthritis and joint degeneration.

I suppose my biggest fear regarding fitness is the inevitable declining cycle ahead. Now more than ever, the support of a good fitness coach is paramount in creating a proactive and comprehensive program.

In 2006, I trained with the vision quest of solo riding the ultimate off-road endurance race. The BAJA 1000. I approached an ex-Air Force trainer versed in aggressive cross-fit style training and during the following year, I gained much strength and cardio capacity.

Pushing at 70-80% for extended periods of time was becoming more and more possible. However, the intensity and pure attack of the training were bringing a whole new host of small injuries beginning to compound. This method of training, although extremely effective, was simply not sustainable for me and my "high mileage" body.

Being flexible in my routine has been paramount in establishing consistency. There are just some days that pain inhibits me from performing certain moves.

At that point, the goal must broaden from getting a specific body part trained that day to simply getting some productive training done that day. Training with an emphasis on physiology, core strength and mobility. This goes back to what kept me off the operating table in my mid 20's and still yields the same dividends 25 years later.

My family is really my primary motivator for staying healthy and mobile as possible. Being an active outdoor adventure crew, my wife and daughters are always looking forward to the next ski trip, or paddle boarding vacation, or mountain biking exploration, or hiking trip.

I suppose what I think of most while training are the many fond memories I have of sharing these experiences with my girls, while imagining all that has yet to come. We often say, "We've got a lot of trail to hit!" The way I frame achievement has morphed and changed so much over the years.

At this time in my life, I believe for me, the ultimate achievement I can hope for is to be active and well for my wife and kids. To make sure my daughters understand what an amazing gift a healthy functioning body is and how important it is to take care of it in a completely comprehensive way.

To set an example with a love for adventure and rising to life's challenges while not letting fear and doubt unduly influence my decisions. Despite my best efforts and intentions, there are days that due to my rap-sheet list of injuries and surgeries, I cannot walk, none the less train.

These periods are disheartening. During one occasion, my trainer, fitness mentor, and dear friend, Michael Parker, sent me this passage that still gets me choked up:

"I am the master of my pain. I am the master of my body. I know and respect my limits. I will strive to be the best I am able, even if less than before. I am my best every day."

I put this up on the wall in my gym with these instructions:

1. Get up
2. Say the words
3. Do the work

This motivates me every day. Every day.

RYAN'S COACHING NOTES

Ryan is one of those people who hit life activities hard from a young age and many of these activities held inherent risks. His level of injury had accumulated quickly compared to most of us, and this exposed the need for structured and deliberate fitness therapies to allow him to mitigate pain and continue his sport.

He was facing a tough decision regarding the potential of spinal fusion because that would alter his capacity for activity for the rest of his life. Ryan learned the value of maintaining a fit body and between his hard work in the gym and added caution, he has continued riding motorcycles to this day.

Fitness is a journey and sometimes we must experiment prudently to find what is right for us at the time. The heavy lifting and boot camp style training has a place, but after a while, it can cause more damage than it is expected to help you avoid.

Ryan was paying attention to his biofeedback and realized he would need to be flexible in his training approach. This is true for anyone with injuries, medical conditions, or suffer from extreme deconditioning. Consistency coupled with the right training approach are key to fitness success no matter your goal.

Ryan has also perfectly tied external factors such as his family activities to his primary intrinsic motivation. This is a powerful way one can separate the intention of fitness from a strictly aesthetic outcome into a functional and purposeful one.

Ryan says it best when he pointed out, "To set an example with a love for adventure and rising to life's challenges while not letting fear and doubt unduly influence my decisions." Fear is a paralyzing agent and can be a constant added struggle for those with injuries to maintain their fitness initiatives.

There are days when Ryan simply cannot get his body to function agreeably and must be extra vigilant in the quality of movement during workouts.

Ryan is inspiring to me personally because I share many of his passions for the outdoors and motorcycling. I also have my own list of injures accumulated over the years as well and must contend with days my body fights back with pain or a newly damaged body part.

Fitness program consistency can be severely compromised by injury or illness and the only way to overcome these situations is to never give up. Ryan is an excellent example of a person who lives life to the fullest by his definition and despite pain, faces each new day eagerly and with joy.

Over the years, I have rarely met anyone so active and concerned about the fitness level of his whole family. Ryan leads the way by mountain biking nearly every single morning before most people are even out of bed.

He gets his corrective exercises and primary lift sessions in daily to whatever degree his body cooperates. He works hard to provide for his family with long hours on the job plus side projects to add extra income.

He gets his family involved in a variety of physical activities and never allows fear or injury permanently stop him from maximizing his life. He does all this despite high-level chronic pain and lots of workout modifications.

For a man so defined by his physical abilities, Ryan has kept such a positive attitude in front of his children even in times of great pain. Yet, I know firsthand it is difficult for him and in private, he can get frustrated, discouraged, and depressed.

Look at the title he chose for his story. To the rest of us, Ryan is such a great example of overcoming challenges and persevering through pain. To him, he sometimes feels broken down because he can recall how he used to perform.

Not for long, though, because he will always rally his mindset and is working hard to be his best every day. He is just as good if not better in his 50's than he was in his 20's. Not because of his athletic ability, but because of his heart and attitude. Where most people give up, Ryan shows up.

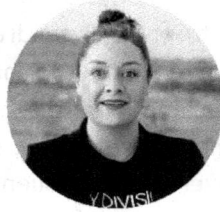

SARA BRADY
"I Was My Own Worst Critic"

I am a 31-year-old senior graphic designer, wife, and a mother of one, currently living in Saudi Arabia. I came to Saudi Arabia originally because of my husband; he works as a researcher in a science and technology university, and sometimes researchers are on a constant move from one country to another. My heritage background is as a melting pot of cultures, from Mexican to Irish American.

My unique heritage history has set my food preferences to my eating habits. From eating until I am stuffed to having my mom say you need to eat everything that is on my plate as a Mexican mom would. I love to paint, bright, and upbeat colors are my game; painting has empowered me to express my feeling, and sometimes my worries about the future in a way that words could not.

I had gone through a long, violent, and toxic relationship since the 6th grade; the only problem was I could not get away from this person. This person has been in my life forever, it's all I have ever known.

And deep down, I loved this person, but it was always a love-hate relationship. The person I was so in love with would physically and mentally abuse me for years to come. Most of my teenage years, I felt alone and depressed, I got bullied because of my weight, and the worst thing is this person also bullied me into thinking I was ugly and worthless. But still, I loved this person, I knew this person could change somehow.

By the end of my senior year in school, I got the worst migraines ever. I had millions of tests done to determine what was wrong with me. No surprise, my prolactin, and thyroid hormone levels were off the roof. This mainly explained my migraine, mood swings, depression, and weight gain, among other symptoms.

Doctors said they couldn't really diagnose me with anything concrete but that I should take some hormonal pills, just in case. After beginning the prescribed medicine, I lost a lot of pounds. I was ecstatic, I was finally skinny! Yet this person still did not love me the way I deserved.

I am currently still living with this person. You might be wondering who this person is? It is ME. Yet I never gave up on me even when I was my own worst critic. I knew I would never be skinny, but I knew there was a better version of me out there.

I concluded this once my purpose in life shifted when I saw for the first time my baby girl's face. I knew that being a woman in this superficial world we live in would make her compare and doubt herself, and I would never want her to struggle the way I have.

This is my biggest fear, and this made me want to change, and I couldn't do it if I didn't change the outlook on myself first. I didn't want to give up on myself and set an example of defeat to my child. Of course, life isn't effortless, and I am still presented with challenges along my journey. I often compare myself with others and forget that I have my own unique setbacks. I live with PCOS; this is one of my hurdles I have to get by every day, and it's a struggle. Sometimes I need to check up on myself and regain my focus on my goal. To be the best version of me I can.

First, I tried most diets and exercises routines that did not help with my PCOS situation. I have tried most fad diets, to name a few, meal replacement shake diet, cabbage soup diet, liquid diet, blood type diet, 3-day diet, you name it, and I have probably tried it.

Now, as far as workouts and classes, I found that my body did not respond well to stressful exercises like Bootcamp and Crossfit. As my stress hormone cortisol rises, I eat more and go into flight or fight mode. I've even exercised to complete exhaustion in one part of my life, and once I didn't see results, I would give up and try the newest workout trend.

The solution is... information, information, information! Once I understood what PCOS is and how my body reacts to different food types and exercises, I started to find strategies to manage my weight. I am learning to have a better relationship with food and how I use it to fuel my body for energy.

I am in a constant learning curb to make better food choices and control my portions, not going to lie once an I while fall stray from my goals, but I have learned two of the greats skill that comes with time and positive thinking.

Perseverance and resilience. You might think they are the same, but they are not. Resilience is defined as "An ability to recover from or adjust easily to misfortune or change" and Perseverance is defined as "The continued effort to do or achieve something despite difficulties, failure, or opposition."- Jerry Scher. Hey, we are not perfect! We learn every day.

My secret is to remind myself that I can be a better version of myself and that my family has a great history of illnesses that could affect me if I don't make a change.

I set goals at the beginning of the day, start with small, realistic, and achievable goals. After a few days, set a more challenging goal, I do this to not discourage myself; once you set crazy goals and you don't achieve them you go rouge, trust me I have been there.

Don't promise something that you will not do. How many of us haven't said I will start exercising and eating healthier tomorrow? And you end up never doing it. Or the typical phrase, I deserve this besides! It's just one piece of cheesecake and it won't hurt, but we end up eating half a pie. Listen, I still go through that. But the key is to change it as soon as you catch yourself going off track.

I have almost completed a whole year of continuous workouts and continue to do so to this day. Keep moving, it's vital for me and makes me feel better and more energetic. It helps me see how far I have come from not being able to do a simple push up to finishing a 5k run in the morning. I am proud of my achievements, however, sometimes, I have to look back to really see the progress I have accomplished.

Remember: Set small goals first; once you achieve them, move on to another one, always challenge yourself. This will keep you on your feet. Never compare yourself; the only competition you should be in is with yourself.

Check-in with yourself, we always give love to others, but we should never forget about ourselves. If at first, you don't succeed, dust yourself off and try again. Failure is a learning tool; it's a chance to try something new. Do this for you!

Think about how this is going to change your life for good or bad, depending on your choice. Be consistent; when the going gets hard, remember why you started this journey in the first place.

Last but not least, reconcile your relationship with yourself first; this will help you along your journey to heal from self-image issues, and to grow into a confident and help repair your self-esteem.

SARA'S COACHING NOTES

Sarah speaks for so many of us that struggle to keep our own self-criticism and internal conversations positive. We can be quite skilled at tearing ourselves down and seeing only the negative and reinforce feelings of defeat through subconscious negative self-talk.

Sadly, this can happen at a young age and we carry the consequences of this throughout our lives if we do not proactively address it.

For Sarah, hormonal imbalance only added to the frustration and feelings of inadequacies, yet she made several important changes to her attitude. But again, she still struggled to reconcile her past reinforced negativity with the reality of finally decreasing bod fat.

Sometimes, we need an external catalyst for change and for Sarah, it was the birth of her daughter. I am an advocate for finding motivators outside of one's self or weak motivators based purely on a superficial aesthetic. I encourage all my clients to find deep personal purpose for remaining healthy and Sarah was able to do that even before we met.

After several months of working with Sarah, I became concerned about the slagging pace of fat loss based on her excellent exercise adherence and food management. I mentioned this to her on a coaching call and a few weeks later, she informed me she was just diagnosed with PCOS.

Immediately, I understood what was happening and I even made significant changes to some of her workouts to keep cortisol levels down and we addressed food quality. I knew Sarah would find her success because her response to the diagnosis in paraphrase was, "Ok, well, it will be slower, but we can do this."

Her resilience and desire to act as a role model for her children despite her own internal battles and physiological complications is incredibly inspiring. Sarah has fundamentally improved how she eats, exercises and views her progress. She is dedicated and even when we hit a roadblock, like this COVID-19 gym closure measure, she perseveres.

Sarah also has it right by setting reasonable goals and personal boundaries she can add accumulative success. I always look forward to the daily photos of her food and portion sizes because this woman eats art. She loves to make beautiful presentations of her food and her ability to add verity is remarkable. One point critical to make is she never lies to herself or me about her food and this is improving her relationship with it.

Sarah also says it best with "Never compare yourself; the only competition you should be in is with yourself. Check-in with yourself, we always give love to others, but we should never forget about ourselves."

This is so powerful because you cannot perform optimally as a partner, parent, employee, entrepreneur or otherwise if you do not take care of yourself. In addition, your journey is your own and comparing your results, body type or any other subjective measure is unadvised.

Compare yourself to yourself. Are you better today than you were yesterday? If not, change it as you have the power and responsibility, just like Sarah.

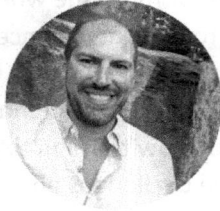

PETER FRIDDLE
"My Best Me"

I have always had an interest in fitness and nutrition. In my early 20's, I found running and that blossomed into a real passion for all endurance sports, including triathlon and long adventure racing.

I guess you could say I had become a weekend warrior, of sorts. I enjoyed competing almost every weekend and naturally stayed fit as I prepared for my chosen sport. In 2015, I went through a very difficult divorce.

My life changed significantly and my time, ability and desire were all waning. I changed careers and started anew with a fantastic company. My new role required a lot of travel and had a fast-paced schedule, leaving little time to focus on wellness.

After a couple of years, I married again, blending two families in two different states. While I wouldn't trade my life for anyone's, I needed to find a new way to integrate self-care, exercise, and wellness into the equation.

The catalyst for action for me came when I realized that I wanted and needed help to find the balance between frenetic and productive. There comes a point where life becomes a series of actions, one to the next. Wellness, as I define it, is the ability to find the center. It allows me to know that I'm taking care of my body and mind, preparing me for the challenges ahead.

It puts life and work into perspective, helping to focus on what is important and helping to shed that which is not. The feeling of being pulled around, for me, happens when I lose my focus on my health and wellness.

That's where I was five years ago. I'm blessed to have found several ways that helped me to maintain and develop a new outlook as I ventured along my wellness journey.

My biggest fears and challenges fall into two general categories. First, as we all are, I am my own worst critic. Never being satisfied and never celebrating success can be a very damaging mindset.

It drives us to abandon what is working because we don't measure up to some artificial image that we've created for ourselves. I have to purposely tell myself to enjoy the journey and to find positive ways to mark progress.

Second, I really enjoy a good meal. I like salty foods, I have a sweet tooth, and I love a perfectly dry glass of red wine. My list of food dislikes is pretty short. Just don't give me a water chestnut.

It's very easy for me to rationalize having the treat. It doesn't take too much inattention for the occasional to become the regular and I find myself back in a place I don't want to be.

I've read and studied lots about exercise and nutrition. I would love to find that magic pill that gives you washboard abs while eating pizza, drinking beer, and watching TV. However, I haven't found it yet, but not for lack of searching.

I've tried a few of the restrictive diets, but I just can't stay committed, especially when travelling and eating in restaurants for multiple meals every week. I have also tried just winging it and that doesn't work either.

Generally, "eating healthy" for me means that certain indulgences creep in until they're a bigger portion of the total than they should be, requiring a course correction. On the exercise side, I like variety. But what I have found is that self-guided weightlifting and training is boring, for me.

I don't know enough to design a program that varies properly, so I either get bored or demotivated, or both. Doing anything with no way to measure progress or compete lacks a point and I quickly plateau and find it hard to push through progress when things get hard.

For me, the formula is simple, yet not always easy to implement. With food and nutrition, I need to focus on eating high-quality foods and on getting enough protein in my diet. This means I need to track calories and be honest about all those seemingly on-off choices I am making that are sabotaging my ability to reach my goals.

With exercise and fitness, what works for me is the realization I need help and support. I need a coach that helps me to design a program. But I also need that coach to help with support and accountability along the way.

I need someone that designs a workout that is harder or longer or different from what I would choose on my own. I need a cheerleader that helps me to recognize progress and to celebrate success.

Keeping motivated is a daily challenge. I have found that the key is to find a system, a process, a way of life that works for YOU. I have taken tips, tricks, ideas, and thoughts from many people I admire and continue to put them together in a way that helps me to stay motivated.

Here are three that come to mind that have served me well. Immediately get out of bed in the morning. Whatever is on your plate for the day, you'll face with more energy and confidence.

Opening your eyes and having a positive thought about your day, followed by immediately getting out of bed to tackle it, has made an incredible difference in my life. The snooze button steals so much more than nine minutes. Surround yourself with positivity.

Work with a coach that gets you and knows how you like to be supported. Figure out how to do this with your spouse. It does not have to be the same, but its sure nice when things can intersect in a positive way.

Compliment others and their progress and see how much better you feel about yourself. As much as possible, keep the food in your house clean. Save the indulgences for what they should be, which is the occasional treat. Healthy snacks and high-quality proteins should be the go-to's at home.

I am on what I am calling the second phase of my fitness journey. Fifteen years ago, I found endurance sports and all that they could offer. I ran a dozen marathons, I ran countless races and I completed an IronMan triathlon.

I found incredible joy and satisfaction in all of those things. However, now my motivation and inspiration are in different places. My achievements are internal and perhaps more subtle.

I'm inspired by my own ability to stay centered and focused in this crazy world. I'm happy when I can recognize and celebrate the progress that I've made. Don't get me wrong; I love hitting a new personal record on the bench, seeing change in body composition, or running a 5K faster than I did a month ago.

But now, it's more than that. It's preparing and eating a healthy meal with my wife. It's working out or taking a walk together with the kids. It's talking about successes and challenges with friends and family, knowing that some of what I shared can help them in their individual journey.

My words of encouragement are simple. Love yourself. The temptation looms large to surround yourself with negativity – you're too fat, too old, too slow, too "insert your own criticism." All of that is completely wrong.

When other people look at you, they see a beautiful person, someone for whom they care very much. Do this for you. Not because anything is wrong or broken, but because we can all be better versions of ourselves.

Treat this exactly as it should be treated – a journey on a road to an inner happiness and joy that you've never experienced before. The power of a healthy body and mind to transform the rest of your life is undisputed.

Your work, your marriage, your relationships will all improve as you navigate through all of the challenges ahead. Don't expect perfection, but don't settle for anything less than your best self

PETER'S COACHING NOTES

Peter is another great example of a person that enjoyed activity in his youth but became distracted with developing adulthood and responsibility. Finding a balance between career, family and personal wellness is a major challenge for most of us.

Peter had some early advantages as he was fascinated by fitness and took the time to educate himself, which most people do not do. In our personal wellness, balance is the product of boundaries. These guidelines are not only the ones we set for ourselves, but also the boundaries we set for employers and family.

It is easy to compartmentalize our lives into separate silos, but this is a mistake related to fitness and nutrition management. For example, folks will silo off their family from career and even fitness from nutrition. This lack of exclusivity creates a fracture in our lifestyle that may not be recognized, but over time, the consequences become evident.

We must create exclusivity in our lives, and this can be defined by boundaries that flex where needed but there are no walls between wellness, career and family. You cannot properly take care of others if you do not tend to yourself first.

I understand this is challenging for many of us, but there are only two options. One is to ignore your wellbeing and constantly self-criticize your physique or performance and remain dissatisfied.

The other option in to make wellness a foundational principle in your life in conjunction with career and family and enjoy satisfaction from the union. Peter has had to elevate his wellness consciousness even higher because traveling causes consistent disruptions with workout type and food quality.

He has had to increase his mindfulness about choices when he has a disruption to keep on track and he has done a great job with this.

One personal discovery Peter made by increasing his wellness consciousness was the ability to identify areas that trip him up. Through some trial and error with fad diets, intuitive eating and workout modes he has discovered what works and does not work for him.

He narrowed down effective ways to align how he approached his unique fitness needs by being objective. Peter also has earned a great deal of knowledge through his studies on fitness and nutrition and has had to learn to resist selective knowledge.

In habit formation and habit alteration, several resistances to change can manifest. One of these is selective knowledge, which is the application of fitness or nutrition information you like, not necessarily what is correct. Peter cleared the clutter and sought help with the formation and progression of his workouts and add a support system for his overall wellness.

I suspect he was applying selective knowledge on his own and found it unsuccessful and boring. For years, I have been honored to work with him and watch his strength rival his incredible endurance. Mostly, Peter thrives on feeling accomplished in his workouts or efforts and when this was written, he had completed over 600 workouts with me.

One note on Peter I feel worth sharing is that his physiological reaction to exercise is not typical. Meaning he really struggles to lose body fat and we have had to be extraordinarily creative to get responses and adaptations. We use a highly structured plan that undulates acute variables in a progressive manner to constantly activate the General Adaptation Syndrome.

This means we apply calculated stress in sets, repetitions, tempo, load, frequency, intensity, total volume and rest to get his body to respond. His strength and endurance are incredible, but compared to most people, the body fat loss is slower.

I felt this was a critical piece for you to understand because despite the slower progress Peter sees in his aesthetic results, he never gives up. He has worked awfully hard to improve his attitude about where he is related to composition and bodyfat and keep chipping away.

Make no mistake, it still is a source of frustration for us both, but no matter what, Peter hits every workout and has recently seen some noticeable composition change despite the COVID-19 situation. Peter is focused on the mindset of becoming the best version of himself and instead of focusing on the result, he is enjoying the journey. I am blessed to be part of it.

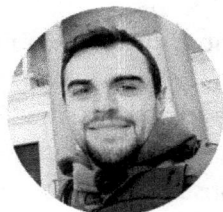

JAMES GRANAHAN
"Skin in the Game"

I come from a small town on the east coast of Ireland and growing up, I always loved sports – playing them, watching them, you name it. I was the kind of kid who always had a ball at my feet and went looking for others to make up teams and play a game. Admittedly, I was never especially much good at sports, but I loved them, nonetheless. However, as I entered my teenage years I played less and less.

I was always quite small – only about 5'9 and not strong or well built – and as sport became more competitive in my teenage years, I dropped away from it. By the time I began college, I had stopped playing sports entirely.

It was by accident rather than intention but nonetheless, I was no longer doing much regular, intensive exercise. I stayed healthy by walking a lot, to and from college, for example, but I was far from fit!

In the years that followed, things only got worse. When college became stressful, I ate more junk food. And with little or no exercise in my routine, I quickly put on weight. I never got fat, per se, but the extra pounds definitely got me down. I'd never put on weight as a kid.

I was always one of those kids who could eat all day and it made no difference. But now, in my early twenties, I could see that my metabolism would not stay like that forever. This extra weight motivated me, and I began to try and exercise again.

For the first time, I consciously decided to go out running and take up yoga. The results were positive, and I often managed to shed a few pounds quickly, but I was never especially consistent, and I soon undid all my hard work.

Fast forward a few more years and the cycle repeated itself again and again. I exercised sometimes, and my nutrition wasn't horrific. But it wasn't good either and I got sick of settling for "just ok".

I decided I wanted to feel good, healthy and strong. More importantly, I saw that I could get away with my bad habits in the short run but that if I didn't change something, I'd end up at 40 or 50 being woefully unfit and probably not very healthy. Ultimately, this motivated me to make a change. But I realized I needed some support.

For years I'd experimented on and off with different exercise and nutrition plans, but when I had to do it all myself, I could never stay accountable. I didn't know the first thing about fitness, so walking into a gym felt scary and intimidating.

I didn't know how the machines worked and I felt stupid. The only thing I knew to do was go running or swimming. But even then, my cardio fitness was woeful, and I found myself stopping and starting constantly, silently suffering through the pain and frustration.

Next, I tried fitness apps. These helped a little bit – at least I had some instructions to show me how to do the kinds of basic gym and bodyweight exercises I'd never tried before. The problem was these exercises varied in level and length. Sometimes they were easy, other times much too difficult.

And worst of all, I didn't even know if I was performing the movements correctly. I had no way of checking my form or getting feedback. And again, the biggest problem of all, was accountability. I had no one there encouraging me and holding me accountable on my fitness journey.

I wasn't motivated because I was simply following a generic exercise plan on an app and I didn't know if it would work for me and my fitness goals. Plus, because I was using these free or really cheap mobile apps, I didn't really have any "skin in the game". I was interested in getting fitter, but I wasn't truly "invested" in it just yet. That would soon come.

In January 2017, I made my fitness a priority once and for all. I was sick and tired of inconsistent efforts and half-baked solutions that didn't make any long-term impact on my health and well-being. That's when I decided to find a coach.

After a few weeks searching, I came across Michael and Forge PT. What drew me to forge was Michael's no B.S. approach to fitness - how he's encouraging but honest – and the idea of having a custom-designed training plan I could show up and follow every day.

I also travel a lot and so I need a lot of flexibility in my workouts and Michael offered this. I'll admit it, the first few weeks were tough! I really wasn't very fit and even the simple workouts I began with hard work at the time.

Looking back, it's kind of funny, really. What made the difference was that I was much more motivated and invested in my fitness now that I had some "skin in the game" and the support of a thoughtful and knowledgeable coach to help me out.

It also became much easier to work out consistently when I didn't have to rack my brain every day, trying to decide what kind of workout or exercise to do. That's the real beauty of working with an expert coach.

You can trust them to build a rock-solid plan designed to give you exactly the results you're aiming for. And you have only to show up and follow that plan. It saves a lot of the mental energy and willpower!

Within a few months, I had completed my first 10km. In less than a year, I found myself in Patagonia, taking on the hiking holiday of my dreams. Just 1 year earlier, I would have really struggled to get around any of the routes.

But with a year of quality training behind me, I knocked out around 100km in just 4 days and one of those was a rest day! Best of all, it didn't even feel particularly difficult. I was fit enough to be able to really enjoy it and appreciate the beautiful nature around me every step of the way.

I think the key to staying motivated is to have a clear goal in mind, ideally something that's not too far on the horizon. One of my best periods of workout completion was in the lead to my first 10km race, because I knew that I'd only be able to complete the race if I diligently showed up and trained each day.

At the time of writing, I'm planning for a long, 12-day hike in the Peruvian Andes and again, having a clear and exciting goal on the horizon has really helped focus my mind during my workouts.

Completing my 1st 10km was a major milestone for me. To have gone unfit and easily out of breath to completing a 10km race within only 7 months was a major achievement and a memory I cherish. I can still remember standing there at the finish line, smiling to myself and soaking in the moment.

It really was an important achievement for me and marked a point where I believed for the first time that with dedication and training, I can take on any physical challenge I set my mind on.

Perhaps more importantly for me, during my first few months of training, I gradually shifted my mindset and personal belief system. I went from being unfit and unhappy with my physical condition to a person who values fitness, nutrition and health. Being fit and healthy is part of my identity and personal belief system now in a way it wasn't before.

I'd encourage people to think about what they want their life to be like – not just today or tomorrow, but 1 year, 5 years and even 20 or 30 years from now. If you want to be mobile, active, fit, healthy and enjoying life fully, then you have to get a handle on your fitness and nutrition. When you're fit and strong, you can take on any challenge. When you eat well and are healthy, you have the energy you need to chase your dreams and enjoy your life.

But it all starts with good daily habits. If you could work out even 2 or 3 times every week instead of ignoring exercise altogether, imagine the difference that would make during a lifetime? Our health and fitness play a major role in the length and quality of the lives we enjoy, so we can't really afford NOT to look after them.

JAMES' COACHES NOTES

James describes a common situation where sports and activity played a role in youth but dissipates over time. We all experience life transitions and one of the most disruptive if from High School to College and then College to Career. We often fail to prioritize our fitness and food management because the consequences are delayed and slowly accumulate.

Our wellness becomes a low priority as we face the reality of family, career and other demanding aspects of life. The lack of attention paid to wellness practices leads to developing unfavorable habits and this new automation reinforces our decline.

Now take these bad habits or diminished fitness and combine that with a lack of confidence or knowledge about how to correct and you have a common picture. Many people struggle to sift through the overwhelming content available related to fitness and nutation. We often get sucked into gimmicks or fads that produce little return or worse, we go through constant cycles of regression.

James made a good go of it on his own but in the end, became frustrated and discouraged. He proactively sought solutions that fit his need and consciously decided to prioritize his overall fitness. In his case, finding a support mechanism accommodating to his specific needs made sense and for over three years, I have had the pleasure of working with him.

Initially, most of James' workouts were considerably basic as we had to start in a progressive manner because of his history of low activity. We focused on connective tissue health, mobility, integrated strength and light cardio work.

Because James deliberately decided to make a personal improvement, he already overcame one of the biggest challenges, which is our own bad attitudes or limiting beliefs about exercise.

Over time, he made considerable improvements in his performance and we integrated complex lifts and advanced running work. James travels often so we would modify his workouts and goals based on what was realistic. In Bulgaria, we had lots of equipment, so strength training was a major focus. In Greece, we did not have that kind of equipment, so we swapped to interval training and running.

James not only improved his physique and strength but ran a good pace in an official 10k. After that, James was bit by the hiking bug, and we worked with cardio conditioning and long-distance endurance.

This allowed him to integrate hiking into his lifestyle and enjoy some remarkable experiences in the outdoors. Mostly, James had a dramatic shift in his own perception of capacity and has incorporated fitness into his inclusive self. Like he says. "...it all starts with good daily habits."

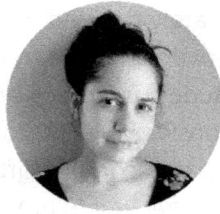

ERICA GUCCIARDO
"Defying My Own Expectations"

I'm a 28-year-old, 4'11" woman who has lived her life in New York and New Jersey, found the love of my life in college, and am now married, a homeowner, and cat parent.

I am a software engineer with a passion for exploring ideas and creating experiences with other people. Though I have trouble being in the moment sometimes, I can always find time to slow down and enjoy my favorite activity - eating delicious food!

During my life there have been many events that slowly pivoted me toward starting a health and fitness journey. The biggest one who comes to mind is my Crohn's disease I've had since I was 9 years old.

Having Crohns throughout my childhood and adolescence was a struggle. Dealing with fatigue and physical pain often deterred me from doing activity - and my proclivity for pursuits of the mind kept my sedentary in my hobbies and career choice.

I've had to learn how to manage my health and be conscious as a result, but this meant scheduling doctor's appointments and complying to medication prescriptions. I've had a handful of surgeries, including one major bowel resection when I was 15 years old.

Crohn's has held me back in many ways, but I've always overcome and come out on top. And I saw it intertwined with my overall health and my future. Given that from a young age, health always had to be a priority, I felt there was one area in which I was always lacking which was my fitness and nutrition.

Another factor on this axis was watching my parents struggle with the consequences of being overweight. Not only them, but many adults. It seems like having weight gain over the course of years seemed almost inevitable, but this is something I wouldn't want for my future. I'm already at a higher risk of more health issues because of Crohns, which also has extra-intestinal symptoms like joint pain.

I felt I even couldn't keep up with my husband when we were first dating and skiing. I was so weak and lacked endurance, muscle, or any sort of precision or flexibility in my movements. I sometimes found it difficult to walk up the stairs and open doors. I knew I was physically weak, and I knew over time this would only get worse, not better.

However, the truth is, from the youngest ages of 12-13, I was getting self-conscious about my body. I held this self-consciousness throughout my life ever since. I would often be on the high end of healthy BMI and occasionally become overweight.

I loved to eat with abandon, especially decked out sushi rolls or a giant 16oz steak, and I often turned to food for emotional reasons.

In fact, I would get such a rush of dopamine every time I ate something I genuinely loved, I would often spend all my time thinking about nothing but my next meal.

I also lay couch-locked for hours and hours each day. I never liked moving my body - it didn't feel good. My Crohn's disease at times led me to unintentionally losing a lot of weight while being very sick, and I noticed one silver lining during these times - I had a lower BMI and, as a result, felt more confident and self-assured. My body shape tends to store excess fat in my upper body - especially my stomach - so the only time I ever felt confident was when I was sick.

However, being healthy came at the cost of me gaining weight - a lot of it - and then suffering from depression as a result of this. I couldn't win. This felt deeply wrong to me. But it also demonstrated to me something that was basically true - all the signs in my life were pointing me in the direction to overhaul my lifestyle and habits.

There are countless examples of the struggles I've had. I probably felt "finally healthy" in 2017, but even before this, I had to learn a lot of difficult skills - such as transitioning from eating out for most of my meals in college to cooking most of my meals once I was on my own. But at the time, I wasn't focused on calorie content.

I also had a lot of mindset issues. I just didn't WANT to change. I didn't want to change my lifestyle, I enjoyed being lazy. I didn't want to change my eating habits, I enjoyed food. I started and stopped countless times with exercise and counting calories. It just couldn't stick. I'd get bored. The novelty wore off. I just couldn't find myself interested.

There was something else more important, like buying my house or interviewing for a new job or working a ton of overtime for a work project or getting a cat. I just couldn't sustain focus for long enough to make concentrated change. The biggest issue was with how I viewed myself.

I viewed myself as lazy and incapable of moving my body for more than 15 minutes. I hated walking. I thought I liked bike riding, but then I wouldn't be able to walk for days. I'd give it my all when skiing and then be in the worst pain of my life. Every time I tried to do something well, it backfired.

It's hard to say what didn't work for me - but not fully committing myself to anything didn't work for me. In contrast to years of on and off exercising - which would come at the cost of being sore for days after the fact - I'd find myself even more downtrodden than ever.

I would try to count calories, but get extremely overwhelmed when I needed to count 10 ingredients in a healthy soup and wouldn't know how to calculate the portions; I'd become frustrated with the tediousness of counting and be good for 2 weeks but then give up in favor of "I don't care that much about losing weight, it's too hard!." I didn't believe in myself.

I found something that temporarily worked exceptionally well for me when I decided I needed to drop weight for my wedding. Here my motivation was the thousands of dollars being spent on a one-day event and the fear of looking back at my wedding photos and cringing.

I stumbled on the WW program, which luckily was much lower maintenance than calorie counting, and it taught me a lot about nutrition, macros, and caloric density, but without needing a ton of time to spend on the education aspect and specifics.

It developed a bit of an intuition around which foods would add up more quickly and which I could eat more freely. Also, it encouraged me to get in more activity because of the Fitpoints concept. But relying solely on the fear of wedding photos wasn't enough for me to keep the 10 lbs I lost off.

I spent 2 weeks in Italy for my honeymoon and promptly gained all the weight back. And then for the following months after, I could not motivate myself to get back into WW despite trying. I felt hopeless.

I was also in the habit of watching Influencers on YouTube - often with an aesthetic which I have only ever dreamed of for myself - sharing their fitness and nutrition recommendations. I had a newsletter for one and she had been advertising a 1-1 coaching program.

I signed up for this because I was still doing poorly with eating below my TDEE (Total Daily Energy Expenditure) and knowing how to structure my workouts to be effective while also being good for my level - and I was overwhelmed and frustrated with the infinite amount of information and knowledge out there and not knowing what was bogus and what would work for me.

Within the first few weeks before the program began, a lot of materials were shared with me which centered on motivation and self-reflection.

I never had thought about looking at my fitness and nutrition journey with the concept of training your mind, not just following some schedule or routine that was supposed to guarantee success.

These worksheets got me thinking and I also identified how much I relied on food to make me happy. Unfortunately, before the program was able to begin, this coach decided to refund my investment as she feared I may have had a binge-eating disorder based on my messaging with her. This really put me in a bad mindset at first - am I so hopeless that no one could help me?

But I knew for a fact that I was far from hopeless; I was committed, and the concept was solid. Another individual, who was very knowledgeable in areas I am not, who could help guide me and show me the pathway to success - to ease my anxiety, to answer my questions, to give me structure and guidance, and to hold me accountable. I had to ensure this is something I wanted before I dove in.

I spent time journaling why it was so important to me to lose weight and achieve the body I always wanted. Because I love myself. Because I want to feel the confidence I felt when I know I'm doing right by my body.

Because I wanted to ski better. Because I wanted to be around for a long time and be active even as I got older. To be able to hike and scuba and swim and enjoy the varied experiences life has to offer.

The key to keeping myself motivated was not to look not only for my extrinsic motivations but also my intrinsic ones. Though a huge goal was to have a certain look - I knew the bigger motivation was self-love. When I worked out, I saw a difference.

A lift in my mood. A feeling of accomplishment, of purpose, of progress. Of defying expectations - especially my own! I saw a shift in my self-perception. I am not lazy. I am not incapable of physical activity, strength, and endurance.

I don't lack the time or the motivation. I had all the pieces of the puzzle. And I needed a better attitude.

An attitude of "I will do this." Getting started was the hardest. Getting started a second time was a little easier, but still hard. But finding ways to make it easy made it easy. This means not obsessing over every gram of food I eat - not all foods are equal, so not all foods need to be obsessed about equally. Moving my schedule to make time for working out.

Committing and following through - and then looking back and seeing that I'm capable. So long as I commit, I can achieve. Committing is the hardest part, and that all relies on motivation, which I found after self-reflecting and really digging deep into my feelings of unhappiness around my former lifestyle, habits, and looks.

And finally, knowledge. The amount you know only grows with time. So, if you don't know a damn thing initially, you can always learn. You don't need to know everything at once to know enough.

I learned this when I jumped head-first into the decision to transform myself for my lifetime and find sustainable habit and lifestyle pivots to help me achieve my goals.

The biggest milestone I have is when my personal trainer and online coach informed me I was doing exceptionally well with my workout adherence and that he could see the results on our weekly calls. I was in disbelief.

Of course, I knew I was putting in the work, because I had faith and belief it would bring with it results. I pushed myself beyond my excuses that cropped up that made me want to skip a workout - whether it be I was tired and sore, or busy, or spent, or just lazy.

But I really fought these feelings hard and pushed them down. I pushed down the desire to just give up and order pizza. I pushed down the desire to stay on the couch and to get down in the gym.

But having it confirmed by someone who really knew this space in and out showed me I am not just losing weight and I am not just trying out some exercise I will eventually get bored of and give up on.

I am changing my lifestyle. I am enjoying it. I'm having fun. I'm pushing myself beyond limits. The way I have always conceptualized myself has been a lazy weak foodie computer nerd who just wants to take a nap.

But now I saw someone different. A person who defies expectations. A person who won't even let her own preconceived notions hold her back from what she truly wants for herself in the present and the future.

And as my trainer recently said, "a performance athlete", which I think is beyond my wildest dreams but I still step up to the barbell to do a workout I've never done before and keep an open mind. I realized there's a curiosity for all that entails in this physical world.

A curiosity for what my body is capable of - and how this will change my life. A curiosity to find my actual limits - not my conceptualized ones - if they even exist!

But what started as fear, depression, and extreme self-criticism and doubt, transformed into something positive and uplifting. I knew deep down I can do anything I set my mind to. I knew this was no different deep down, but I wanted to avoid facing the work. But now I think back, and I don't know why I was avoiding it. I think if I were to guess it is because I did not realize that over time my self-perception would change.

That I wouldn't just be the lazy, unfit girl flailing in the gym and getting winded in 15 minutes forever. That I wouldn't just be the person who couldn't control their eating and had no idea how many calories they just ate forever. These things faded with time and repetition. Practice makes perfect; I had to learn being perfect isn't a deterrent and that my self-perception was the one holding me back.

I couldn't see myself in the future with a different lifestyle until I did. I sat down and pictured myself in 2-3 years after committing myself fully. I imagined myself as happy, confident, fit, and physically capable of things I never was ever before.

Hell, who would have expected that I started seeing this happen in 1 month of following my workouts consistently? Something as simple as not being able to do a kettlebell windmill on week 1 to them being easy on week 4.

Consistency motivated me because my future became my present - and I worked towards that future every day, closing the gap every day. Finding new possibilities every day. And NEVER letting my doubt become paralyzing. I always tried to externalize the doubt and find another angle to look at it.

This new angle was positive and focused on the possibility and potential if I just persist and persevere and trust that hard work pays off in waves and isn't linear. Whenever you hit the bottom of the wave, know there is another one swelling up and get back up so you can ride it with a giant, self-assured, confident smile.

Look at yourself in the mirror and love yourself for the small differences or for being able to lift more or being less sore after going for a walk or run - these small milestones will add up to larger ones.

I look back at myself in 3 months - only 3 months - and I'm a completely different person. I'm not just someone losing weight for some wedding photos. I transformed my entire lifestyle and my future. And I know I can keep doing things forever.

I know I won't revert because I love the process and journey just as much as I love the results. Being fit had entirely unexpected benefits - my mood is lifted, my energy is higher, and I surprise myself constantly with the results of building muscle.

Lifting more, moving my body more, feeling energized after a workout instead of spent. I look forward to doing things I never did before because of my new lifestyle, and I know that anyone can apply themselves and change their lifestyle through self-reflection, commitment, faith in your own potential, and the belief that the bright future you deserve is possible when you put in the work!

ERICA'S COACHING NOTES

Erica represents a great deal of young women I work with today. From an early age, she became self-conscious of her body but with the added stress of a digestive disease. She was not only working through the insecurities of youth, she was in pain, fatigued and limited in her capacity by comparison.

Erica also observed her family struggling to maintain a handle on their own fitness and nutrition. This can often lead to children growing anxiety around food and learning to fear or devalue exercise.

Like most of us, Erica has some deep emotional ties to food and has worked hard to improve her relationship with it. Unfortunately, she also had to overcome disordered thinking about her illness and how it was causing unhealthy weight loss.

Losing weight from an illness is rarely a positive or healthy occurrence and can lead to further psychological complications that manifest into physical complications. Wellness and the sum of body weight are not necessarily linked. Your total body fat percentage compared to your lean tissue is a healthy and proactive metrics for measuring your fitness success.

One of the most potent parts about Erica's story is when she stated there was no desire for her to make a change. She was at a point where the instant gratification of food and laziness provided higher reward than a fit body and healthy lifestyle. Usually, there are two reasons for this.

First, we are always seeking homeostasis, even if that consistency is negative or has accumulating consequences. Second, the instant gratification has delayed those consequences and we can skim by for a time gaining weight and try to justify our behavior. In the end, we always get caught and must pay for the crimes against our body.

While educating yourself about fitness and nutrition is critical in today's world of easy food access and low activity, when must be careful where we get this information. In my experience, it is almost never from the internet or social media as there are significant misinformation and conflicting opinions. After sorting through this, we must decide what works best for ourselves and apply common sense disciplines, not obsessions or dogma.

It is true, after a time, I told Erica that her programming and performance had moved into an athletic level. She is doing compound moments, structured and periodized workouts, and her composition has improved remarkably with lean muscle and lower body fat.

Yet the most significant changes for her have been attitude and paying attention to habit and the root causes behind her struggles. We address then systematically and with deliberate programming. Now she can work to become even better and over time, she will have mastery over her workouts and food choices.

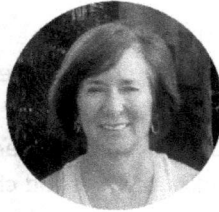

ALI HARRISON
"Be Your Best Self"

I am 62 years old, splitting my residence between Oxford, PA, and Boynton Beach, Florida. I grew up in Silver Spring, Maryland, in the Washington, DC, suburbs. I was a highly active kid, playing kickball, baseball, and other games outside in the backyard with all the neighborhood kids.

When I was three years old, my father started a summer camp for children in the Blue Ridge Mountains of West Virginia. I spent every summer at camp and I grew to love the outdoors, camping, and movement of any kind, whether it was running, a game, or a sport.

I felt free and confident when I was moving, otherwise feeling somewhat shy. Around the age of twelve, when I entered junior high school, I started feeling out of place and from that discomfort emerged even more of a passion for sports and activity. I loved running and was a fast sprinter.

It was through sports that I was acknowledged and found my comfort zone. Around this time, my dad had an opportunity to become the high school tennis coach at the high school where he taught. He bought a book on the mechanics of tennis and we played. As I went to high school, I participated in volleyball, basketball, track, and tennis.

I excelled at most anything athletic. After high school, I traveled to West Chester, PA, to become a health and physical education teacher. Wester Chester was a very well-regarded school in the areas of health and physical education.

Part of being a physical education and health major was participating in a sport at some level. I dreamed of playing basketball or running track. I was one of the few out-of-state students and knew no one from my hometown attending West Chester.

My parents were not supportive of my move out-of-state, and I had to move myself into the dorm. The first two girls I met across the hall from me were trying out for the tennis team and they encouraged me to go with them to the try-out.

I was desperate to make friends, and I really had no intention of playing tennis seriously, but after somehow making the team, I was hooked. I attribute my connection with my teammates and coach to much of my college success. It pointed me in a very positive direction and I had 4 successful years both in tennis and the academic world.

Tennis became my first love, and it was in college that I began my wellness journey. My college tennis coach was the fittest person I had ever met. She ran 5-10 miles every day and encouraged us to become fit.

I started running with her and accompanying her to lunch. I never had a major weight problem, but most likely would have as I got older. I would call myself a little chunky at that time. Having come from short, muscular (dad) parents, I didn't realize at the time that I would be fighting an ongoing battle with my weight.

After beginning to run, my body started to change, and I ate a little less and skipped the potato chips. When I went back to visit my high school tennis coach, he told me I looked fifteen pounds lighter, but I think it was more a fat decrease than a decrease of pounds on the scale. It was here, at college, that I started to become interested in the physiology of exercise and my quest to fight the aging process.

After graduating, I got a job teaching summer tennis and another job teaching physical education in a private school. I loved my like-minded colleagues and I went to the gym or ran with someone from the department every day. This was in the early 80s, where gyms and fitness for women were starting to take off.

I continued along this path, always making my work-out a priority. I then got a teaching job at a public school and my time was more limited. I had a gym membership and lived in the quaint small town where I attended college. I enjoyed running a loop through town. I did the occasional 10k but was never great at long distances.

I had improved through training but was still a much better sprinter. I did love the freedom that running made me feel and before the era of cell phones, I knew I could run somewhere if I was stranded with a broken-down car. I was hard on myself and upset if I missed a workout. I was overly critical of my body.

I had sprinter-like protruding thighs on a 5'2" frame and people either admired them or detested them. What other people thought of me mattered a lot. I had a boyfriend at the time who contributed negatively to my problem and critiqued my physique.

I was in a dysfunctional relationship and found myself depressed a lot. It fed into my lack of confidence, and I remember my late 20s as being one of the worst times in my life. Exercise helped me get through. I hadn't given up on myself completely and tried to do something positive for myself each day.

I finally moved on and met someone who made me incredibly happy. I worked out in some form or another for the next 25 years. In 1999, I married my husband and we moved to a rural area called Oxford, PA. I was a gym member at the local Y for 17 of those years and found that I could only keep up with exercise and work if I got up at 4:50 AM and got over to the gym.

I had an hour commute into suburban Philadelphia and could not get motivated to do anything after work. I skipped workouts and couldn't get out of bed some mornings, but I managed to maintain a better-than-average level of fitness. I was also able to work out in the early morning at the school where I taught.

I would run in the gym or parking lot and sometimes swim in the pool. I continued to play tennis and squeezed it in whenever I could. I played in the USTA (United States Tennis Association) leagues and worked towards my tennis teaching pro certification.

I continued to improve my skills and still believed that I could become a better player. My biggest setback came in my early 50s. I had been playing in the USTA league and training and had started taking a lesson weekly. I was working on improving my volley and felt a sharp pain in my wrist.

I went to see the sports medicine physician, and he told me I would have to give up tennis due to severe degenerative arthritis in my dominant wrist. His bedside manner was gruff, and I came out of his office crying and thinking life as I knew it was over. After the appointment, I talked to a physical therapist I knew, and I asked him about fitness training to try and work around the wrist. He thought it was worth a try.

This was where I began a fitness program in earnest with a trainer. I also worked to improve my tennis techniques. Ten years later, I am managing to play a high level of tennis, better than in previous years, relatively pain-free, and have remained injury-free as well. I worked out with a few trainers sporadically over the years.

I could not afford weekly visits, so my visits took place every couple of months. I would walk away with a workout I could do on my own. Most trainers were not interested in this arrangement and I had trouble finding someone to take me on. That is how I discovered Forge Online Training.

I tried multiple diets and found that the best eating plan for me was one of non-processed foods and calorie restriction. My weight fluctuates and every day is a struggle. My goal now is more to maintain what I have and be happy with who I am. I am not that twenty-something anymore. I am happy with my body and what I have done to keep fit. I discovered that a home gym works well for me. I can make efficient use of the time I have available without adding in travel. Play tennis, and now also golf, burns calories and gives me some great social contacts and is fun!

I am retired so I have plenty of time now to do what I enjoy. I love being able to feel young and able to keep up with my age forty-something teammates. I have forged many friendships through sports. I want to live a long active life and I keep that in mind when I begin to struggle through a workout.

I feel really good most every day and not everyone can say that. I attributed it to trying to maintain a level of health and fitness. It is certainly good for the mindset. I am proud of myself for persevering.

Despite challenges, keeping your goals in the forefront is the way to stay motivated. Just remembering how good you feel when you complete a day, week or a month's worth of workouts. You can feel proud that you are not sitting on the couch, letting age get the best of you.

And you are adding years to your life, and to me, that is the biggest bonus of all! One thing I am most proud of is captaining and playing on a USTA National Championship 55 and over tennis team.

My friends and I worked together for 20 years not only to achieve the goal of advancing to the national championships but actually winning the championship in 2017. It was the best feeling, the most fun, and the greatest sense of camaraderie I can ever remember. We were so happy and proud! It just makes me want to keep going! My goal now is to play tennis into my 70s, 80s, and 90s as I have seen others do.

To inspire others, I have a few suggestions. Start small and try and be consistent. Don't beat yourself up if you miss a day or you don't go as far as you planned. Listen to how you feel. You will have good days and bad days, just try and squeeze in something. Squeeze in a walk at lunch. Make small changes in your diet.

Find a friend that might have similar goals. Motivate each other to stick with it. Get some training help from a trainer (mine is Michael Parker with Forge) and find a nearby gym that suits your needs.

Take classes or use videos. Staying fit has tremendous mental and physical benefits and gets you through difficult times. You can be proud of yourself for just sticking with it.

ALI'S COACHING NOTES

Ali is an outstanding example of a person who connected the importance of physical activity to quality of life early on. While she does mention aesthetics and body composition in her story, she was able to tie intrinsic goals based on performance to her lifestyle. This was further reinforced by a positive influencer who set a strong example.

The power of associating with folks who take their wellbeing seriously can have a profound effect on your own desire or willingness to be active. This is a common theme in her life, and I suspect it is because of her connection to sports and other athletes, along with her own drive.

Yet, even with Ali's strong internal drive and high activity level, she still struggled with all the same things we do. Even though her performance was a prime focal point, she still found physical parts of herself to criticize or disrupt her confidence. Even people that appear to be on top of their fitness still experience frustration, setbacks and dissatisfaction.

It is easy for those people that are constantly starting and stopping a diet plan or fitness program to become resentful. But we all struggle in a similar fashion and instead of jealousy or judgment, we should all strive to make wellness an inclusive part of our lives. It's hard for everyone, even the people who make it look effortless.

I would also point out that she was able to find a proactive way of maintaining her activity in a period of life that was challenging. Even when her work schedule and life situation made it difficult to get to a gym, she still found ways to be active and retain her fitness.

In addition to this, she worked hard to recover from an injury that could have seriously hindered her ability to perform in her sport. I have found two of the most common reasons people quit is when exercise became inconvenient and loses priority or they get injured.

Ali never gave up despite experiencing some of the prime reasons most people simply fail with fitness. She was disciplined and driven to maintain her performance through aging and has had enjoyed outstanding accomplishments because of her dedication.

As she says, you can be proud of just sticking with it and let results be the byproduct of your consistency over a lifetime.

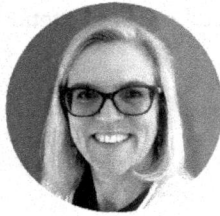

MOLLIE HOLT
"Inattentive to Intentional"

I grew up in a family of goers. We lived in many places as my dad worked for the federal government and was often transferred. My stay home mom insisted we get out of the house for as many hours possible.

During summer, she allowed my three siblings and I to eat breakfast and watch TV through the Price is Right. Then, outside we went. Home for lunch and dinner hours, and home to bed when she flashed the porch lights.

During the school year, we all played organized sports each season. My parents did not care if we excelled; rather, they expected us to meet new friends, be good teammates and get some exercise.

On weekends to give Mom a break, Dad took us adventuring. Hiking, fishing, skiing, sledding – whatever seemed fun outdoors. The entire family ate like horses and remained very fit and healthy. I never learned about nutrition – I ate what mom provided. I never worried about weight – it just was not an issue in our household. I did not appreciate my fitness – it just happened. Until it did not.

Over the years of raising two daughters and working full time as a certified public accountant (long hours of sitting), I found myself incredibly out of shape and overweight. However, due to good genetics, my blood sugar levels, blood pressure and cholesterol remained low. I did not experience any life impeding health issues.

As a result, I could not motivate myself to change. I was too darn busy working and raising my family to make myself a priority. I accepted that I had a belly and bikinis were out of the question.

Then I hit fifty. I noticed that nobody pays attention to a middle-aged, overweight woman. Little things like catching the waiter's eye, being served at a crowded bar, friends commenting on how good I looked, random smiles from strangers when you know you look healthy and fit.

I wore baggy, unflattering clothes to be comfortable. No cute strappy heels as my feet and ankles would swell throughout the day. This was all upsetting, but I had not yet thought a change was necessary.

The tipping point happened at the doctor's office for a regular checkup. All my numbers were up and some of them borderline for medication. I got on the scale (which I had avoided for 25 years) and watched in horror as the nurse kept moving the slider up.

It stopped at 185 pounds. I am 5'5" and small-boned. I faced that I was technically obese. And I had no idea how to fix it. I did not know where to start. I worked a very sedentary, stressful job with long hours.

My coping mechanisms included cooking and eating huge delicious meals with family and friends and frequent happy hour and appetizers with my girlfriends. How could I find time to get fit? But then I came across a quote (I do not know who to attribute it to), "It is very hard to lose weight and get fit. But it is also hard being fat." Bam. My Truth.

My youngest daughter suggested I try Whole 30, a very regimented eating plan with many restrictions on what to eat. I tried and hated it. Lost 20 pounds in a month and put it back on the next. Tried it again with the same results. I tried randomly exercising when I felt the need.

I hit the gym a couple of times a week. I cut carbs. But what was lacking was a PLAN and a GOAL. I needed to hold myself accountable for something that was achievable. And I needed a place to start because it is hard to exercise when you are packing an extra 50 pounds.

It is hard to vision end goals with small steps on the journey. I did some soul searching. I had grown tired of being overweight and unable to perform basic fitness exercises such as sit-ups, push-ups or jumping jacks.

At 52, I knew myself well. My journey would need to be slow, with readily accessible resources that were safe and welcoming (i.e., not the gym and not face to face), and not horribly time-consuming.

I could not handle a trainer yelling in my face, a coach striving to get me to a 5K race nor a regimented plan, which was not feasible with my schedule. I also live in a very small rural town. So, I decided it would have to be online.

My ability to stay motivated is pretty simple. I want to be active and do fun things until I am in the grave. I want to wake surf with my family and friends, go on a bike ride around Lake Coeur d'Alene with a beer and ice cream at the end of the ride.

I want to ride the Hiawatha Trail to the bottom and back up again. I want to cross country ski and hit the lodge for ski appetizers and drinks. I do not want to be the one waiting for others to come back. I don't want to be the one holding up the crowd.

As I started my story, my extended family remains incredibly active and fun. I don't want to be on the sidelines - I want to be participating and enjoying the adventures. This is powerful!

I decided to make this a journey of small steps and victories. I celebrate along the way and enjoy the process at each step. I remember vividly the first time I could do a burpee, get fully into child's pose without my belly in the way, and finish an intense HIIT workout without stopping. I get such satisfaction when moving to the next barbell weight. Dropping a dress size. No swollen feet. Lowered cholesterol. an excellent resting heartbeat.

Each of these small on their own but impactful in my journey. Get your mind right before you try to get your body right. Figure out the whys of being unfit and overweight. Then be real and accept them.

The next step is to commit to attack in a way that works for you. Your journey is not your neighbor's journey. Make it your own. And be easy on yourself if you continue in the right direction. Victories don't happen every day.

MOLLIE'S COACHING NOTES

Mollie hails from a period when being a child was about adventures and the outdoors. I had a remarkably similar upbringing with the level of activity and eating what was put in front of me.

One advantage of youth is the body can be quite forgiving and in the right environments, we crave activity as children. Sadly, we have seen a major social shift with children leading sedentary indoor lifestyles along with an obsessive fixation with electronic devices.

I worry over this because if Mollie, who came from a far more active generation, suffered a negative turning point in her later years, how soon will our children be obese and facing medical consequences for inactivity and ignorance towards food?

The power in Mollie's story comes from the realization that body composition, excess fat, swollen ankles or poorly fitting clothes are not a strong motivator for change. As modern humans, we live in a world of widely accessible calorie-rich foods and lead low activity lifestyles.

Eating is easy and enjoyable, while moderating food and exercising seem less appealing to most folks. In addition, the accumulation of fat and deconditioning is gradual, so the consequences are not immediate and easy to ignore. Yet almost everyone will make a loose goal to "lose weight" now and then but their intention is nearly always about aesthetics.

Unfortunately, we know for a fact that an aesthetic goal is one of the cheapest and low return motivators. This is evident in the exploding rate of obesity in adults and children plus the saturation of fitness products on the market.

The products exist because consumers continue to buy them, looking for a quick fix to a long-term problem. All these products serve to trap people in a never-ending cycle of fitness failure. This is where we start a diet or fitness program only to quit within weeks and return to our normal habits. When we start these programs, our goals are typically about weight loss or a superficial composition outcome.

But soon, pizza becomes more important because you get instant gratification, which sounds more fun than reducing ankle swelling because you can just wear flat shoes or hide your problem in baggy clothing. It is also easy to prioritize the care of others over our own wellbeing, but the bill will come due at some point.

For Mollie, it was the realization that being fat is super hard too. Not only is it difficult, it has nothing but negative consequences for your composition, health and performance. Inevitably, medications are needed to supplement the body's normal functions because we have become so unwell, it can not maintain its own systems without drugs. Let that sink in.

Now we have two powerful motivators exposed for Mollie, which include avoiding medical intervention and improving her performance. She wanted to have an active life and be able to fully participate in these activities, so the excess body fat became an impedance to her intended outcome.

This intrinsic motivator gave her just the right amount of fuel to seek improvement. Most importantly, her attitude changed about why she wanted to get fit and she began to set reasonable expectations based on little victories.

As for composition, Mollie has drastically improved her aesthetics, but they are a byproduct of working on her food management and exercise adherence. She focused on improving her overall wellness in increments and expanded her exercise ability and added all sorts of supplemental activities to her life.

Cycling, hiking and structured workouts make the majority of this and have improved her quality of life. Mollie is a perfect example of someone who decided to change her attitude about fitness and celebrate the journey instead of focusing on a subjective superficial outcome. Now she gets to enjoy the benefits of her hard work in performance and physique and won't be on the sidelines ever again.

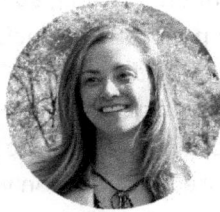

MAILE LONO-BATURA
"Becoming the Best Version of Me"

I have been so fortunate to grow up with incredible backdrops–born on Maui, grew up in Montana and Washington. Growing up swimming (getting plowed by waves) and skiing and snowboarding among the snow ghosts on Big Mountain and the many faces of snow conditions in the Cascade Mountains.

My mother was born and raised in Montana and my father on the island of Maui, so I guess I lucked out being rooted in some prime locations. I'm now raising my own kids along the gorgeous Cascade Foothills of Washington State with my husband, Ryan.

Being connected to and appreciating our surroundings was something I grew up with and wanted my kids to experience as well. I have two kids – Schaller is 12 and June is 3. Neither is very risk-averse, which is both fun and terrifying to watch.

Both with very signature personalities that I couldn't possibly have scripted. I've been with my husband for 21 years and am amazed at how a couple of radicals like ourselves have learned how to function as a family. We love to explore our hiking trails, skateboard, bike and enjoy all seasons of mountain sports.

While our 3-year-old is not quite as mobile and experienced, she comes along with us when possible, so we have experiences together as a family (hint: pack lots of snacks). We love music too – possibly a little obsessively – and it suits us.

Ryan is the lead singer and guitarist in a rock band and I spin tunes as a radio DJ for a local Hawai'i music show. Music is everywhere and our kids are homing in on what they love (and don't love).

For a good majority of my life, my 'exercise' was mainly the sports or activities I was involved in. I wasn't really compelled to workout or even necessarily pay much attention to nutrition – if it tasted good, I'd probably eat it.

It wasn't until I was pregnant with my first child that I realized not only was someone truly relying on me for their health and safety, I would also be a model to them of how they should take care of themselves.

There is one additional reason that prompted my wellness journey, and while I should probably leave it out, I should mention that my husband has an uncanny ability to excel at pretty much any sport he tries.

It's a little annoying and also admirable. It also means my A game is not even near his, so it's been actually healthy to push myself a bit more to at least play in the same league.

Getting Schooled: I've mentioned this to Michael in my training, there is always that level of excitement of what new plan is coming on board, and it is coupled closely with the fear of not being able to do it.

For example, we started a push-up challenge to 'push' myself to do more and see how much I could improve over time. My upper body strength is much better than when I started a year ago, but I was skeptical about how my body would react. Regardless, I tried and got majorly schooled, and that's just a part of the journey.

Injuries: My lower back is pretty finicky, and in the past year, it's gone out a handful of times due to bad lifting technique on my part. There are certain exercises and general movements that I'm just more careful doing now.

Progress: Being pregnant is both amazing and a complete morphing of your body. While I know that I'm making progress in fitness and overall wellness, sometimes it's just hard to see results. I do feel it, though, and that is pretty incredible.

Nutrition: This fear turned out not to be as difficult as I thought it would be. Eating good food pays off in spades, it's just making sure that there are more good calories than empty calories. I continue to struggle with that and finding a way to stay within the lines as best as possible.

Gyms: While the access to all the equipment and amenities is supreme - for me, it became a time and money sink.

Leading with Restrictions: It might just be my personality (my husband would agree), but tell me I can't do something, and I will successfully tune you out. With nutrition and fitness, leading with restrictions instead of outlining goals and what that will lead to is the first step on a short journey.

Home Gym: I can literally walk out to the garage and be in a functioning gym space. It can be a little chilly in the winter, but it motivates me to get the warm-up going.

Videos: Before I had tried exercise videos, I might be a bit skeptical as to their effectiveness. I've learned, though, that if you put a kickass instructor leading you through an exercise routine that you're into, you'll burn calories and have fun. Kickboxing and Pilates are a few of my favorites.

Progress tracking: No lie — it is tedious at times. It is so worth it, though, to see your progress (and regression) and what you can do to manage your nutrition and activity. It essentially puts you in charge so that there is no mystery why your run the following morning might not have been the greatest.

Schedule: For both nutrition and fitness, it has been key to have a schedule to follow as best as I can. For example, if I don't get my workout done in the AM, it probably won't happen. If I don't eat a snack around mid-morning, I will overeat at either lunch or dinner.

Support: My family supports and cheers me on. When I come in from the gym or a run and feel pretty beat, Ryan will let me know how awesome it is that I got it done and how proud he is of me. The support from Forge has been so important to me making these changes in my routine to be a better version of me.

I look forward to checking in with Michael to problem-solve or revise what's on the horizon. And really just having someone there to help guide you through it all. It would be so much more difficult without this support.

Some tips: Go one more if you can. If you slack or fail on a move, do it again and do it right. Believe you can. Remember who you're doing it for. Every workout is a step to becoming a better version of yourself, for you, your family and to represent for those before you.

One of the major sources of inspiration to be my best self, is where and who I have come from. Knowing that I wouldn't even be here to live and nurture myself if it wasn't for the chance happening of being born.

So, it is motivating to me to remember this and that what I think is hard, pales in comparison to what those before me have endured. My Grandparents grew up during a time where it was rare to be sedentary at all during the day.

Fitness was really just doing your part to support your family. In Montana, my Grandma, who is now 98 years old, lived through World War II and the Depression. She worked in a gypsum plant during the war, herded sheep and raised her own family in power stations where my Grandpa worked.

My Grandparents from Maui raised 15 kids (not counting the hippies that also stayed with them) living primarily off the land and ocean. Everyone had a job to contribute to the whole (hippies too), and if you didn't contribute, you didn't eat with the family. They worked hard and yet lived pretty simply without excess and always extending aloha to others in need.

Being a model for my family is as important as representing for those that came before me. It's so easy to say I should workout, I should eat better because the intention alone feels kind of rewarding that you're even considering it.

When I get up and start naming all of the reasons I don't want to workout, I remember to start listing all of the names of people that I do it for, the times that I was unable to lift any weight due to injuries or sickness and all of a sudden, it feels like an honor, not a burden.

It feels like I'm doing this for not just myself – I'm doing it for all of the people I care about and for every day I get to be here.

MAILE'S COACHING NOTES

Maile is an excellent example of how to integrate fitness and nutrition in an inclusive way that not only benefits herself, but also her family. Being active as she is with a career and several children, we can clearly see how she grew to prioritize her fitness despite all the distractions in life.

It did not always start out this way, but with time and experience, she was able to make the connection. When she started with me over a year ago, it was just about snowboard season, and we really focused on workouts that would translate to her favorite sport.

This has become a bedrock approach for all her workouts. We focus on building programs that challenge her ability but also improve her function in sports and recreation.

Like most of us, Maile has had a few small injures and other unexpected issues come up, but we always find a solution and modify to keep her progressing safely. I point this out because what makes this work is her positive attitude and the fact she never gives up.

Her desire to learn about her unique body performance and to improve nutrition has made a big difference in her composition and strength despite injury or pregnancy. She is another great example of how a home gym can be a huge return on investment because she uses it.

Maile is very athletic and capable of some advanced lifting and high-intensity work. She never complains and has aligned her mindset in such a way that the very act of working out brings just as much satisfaction as results.

Tracking is a hard thing for most folks because, as she mentioned, it can be tedious. But she has embraced the power of information and we often use her tracking logs to determine progressions or troubleshoot.

I like to include Maile in the basic outline of her workouts because she is willing to try new movements or push herself to improve her technique. This makes it easier to keep her moving forward and avoid over-long stages of plateau.

The most powerful thing I take away from her story is the inclusion of others in her motivation. She has tied her family in as deep intrinsic motivators, and this helps her overcome the days she just feels like skipping out or ignoring her food consumption.

I strongly encourage all my clients to find these motivators because they will carry you further than superficial motivations like weight loss. Her gratitude for life and the example she sets for her children are inspiring to me.

While she is honored to work hard for them, I am honored to be part of her life and walk with her on this journey.

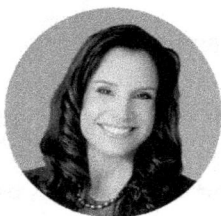

ALEXANDRA STILLMAN
"If You Fall, Get Up and Try Again"

I am a 52-year-old married female. I run my own business as a health and medical psychologist so focusing on my own health and wellbeing has always been a top priority for me. For the past 2.5 years, I have had severe, intractable chronic migraines since my early 20s.

When I hit 49, I entered menopause, which threw me into a whole new category of increased headaches, decreased sleep and mood swings. Prior to this time, I had been athletic running 2-4 miles each day, lifting weights twice a week and doing Pilates/yoga for fun. My nutrition was structured and healthy and I felt great.

Although I have had a fitness focus all my life, my three-primary health and their co-morbid mental health concerns were debilitating migraines up to 25 times per month, myofascial pain syndrome and menopause.

I had been seeing a medical provider who prescribed heavy pain medications and provided few other options.

I was no myself and was clearly overmedicated. I decided to make huge changes in my health and wellbeing. I switched primary care physicians, got off all pain medications and began exploring ways to both manage my symptoms holistically.

I focused on nutrition, exercise and alternative pain management strategies such as physical therapy, neurological interventions, acupuncture and appropriate amounts of rest. I admit I did not have much energy to follow through on these goals until I decided to seek support for both physical and motivational aspects of my health and wellbeing.

I am still relatively new to the Forge program, but between this training platform, meeting with a registered dietitian and engaging in streaming online Zoom classes, I actually feel excited and happy about exercise and nutrition for the first time in years.

Sadly, I am not consistent with much of anything and my motivation waxes and wanes. I find weekly coaching calls with a trainer who is competent in nutrition, exercise and motivation to be the most powerful factor in the changes I have made to date. I have some epic fails I would like to share as a caution to avoid.

First, I tried "fad" anything from nutrition to exercise to sleep gimmicks. Second, forcing myself to work out when my body is genuinely fatigued or lacking nutrients. Third, I have historically struggled with following through on commitments. And finally, I also have had the negative tendency to think of exercise as all or nothing: either I run 3 miles, or I do not go outside at all.

I have learned and am practicing that if you fall, get up and try again. There is no such thing as failing if you are trying. I am now a big fan of listening to my body and reminding myself that moderation and modification are my friends.

I also like using nutrition tracking apps and entering what I plan to eat the next day, so I gave a roadmap. Same things for exercise - the more solid the plan, the more likely it is to happen. I am also a big fan of asking for support and encouragement when I need it. I also find drinking a lot of water makes a dramatic difference in how I feel and function.

Motivation has been and is one of the pieces that has been a larger struggle for me. I use mediation to help change negative thoughts about eating and exercise. I am a huge fan of making plans and then checking boxes for completed goals and monitoring my progress, which is quite easy to do on the Forge app as well as on my nutrition tracking app.

I find the common trick of always laying out my exercise clothes at night for the next day very helpful. I also always keep a laptop in my workout area at home, so it is convenient and meal prep on the weekends.

I ran 2 5ks at 48 and I have asthma and not the body type that is conducive to running. I have also made gains in my eating, eliminating soda and attempting to keep my added sugars to 6 teaspoons a day.

My most important achievements, though, have been mental - I have actually been able to say I love my workouts. I also am experiencing fewer headaches, fewer mood swings and improved sleep.

Point is, don't be so hard on yourself. Any movement or any positive nutritional change is a win. This can look like walking around the block or adding another serving of vegetables a day. I know we all think, "I'm too busy." That is an excuse and a poor choice.

Again, any movement counts whether that is taking the stairs instead of the elevator or taking the far parking spot. Be proud of yourself each and every time.

ALEXANDRA'S COACHING NOTES

Alexandra has worked awfully hard to overcome chronic pain and find ways to improve her overall wellness. Despite relatively consistent setbacks and reoccurring migraines, she never stops looking for a solution.

Her personal philosophy, "There is no such thing as failing if you are trying," is a powerful statement of positive defiance against circumstances out of her direct control. We all have some form of interference in our lives and few of them derail adherence to exercise programs quicker than an injury or pain.

She has examined and is working to reject the "all or nothing" mentality and is celebrating even the smallest success. This is fundamental to recovery in her situation because she has begun to create realistic expectations based on her current condition.

This makes it easier for her to set goals that are a bit of a stretch but are still something she can achieve without exacerbating her issues or causing resentment towards the process. She was also able to identify satisfaction from completing her daily tasks and being able to check-off boxes as complete.

In Alexandra's current training phase, we are working more towards habit development and daily goals focused on meditation, nutrition targets, hydration, and light corrective movements. Over time, we assess her condition and will add intensity appropriately to minimize any potential relapse into pain. Her willingness to objectively examine her state each day and still try for some form of activity is making quite a difference for her. Her renewed excitement towards fitness is reinforced by her small yet significant daily successes and validates her decision to abandon her old psychology of all or nothing. Every little bit adds to the sum of success.

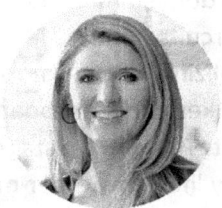

HEATHER TURNING
"Never Give Up"

I grew up home-schooled and an only child. This made life interesting since I had a lot of time on my hands. After my mother left for work in the morning, I stayed home and scheduled out my day. Even though I didn't have a teacher or parent telling me what I had to do with my day, I still felt that I needed structure, so I made my own school lessons and fitness routine.

I eventually came across an exercise tape behind our VCR and made it part of this routine. I would play this wonderful 80's video full of people in tight spandex working both cardio and body weight for an hour. Then, after finishing some homework, I ended up jumping on my bike for hours exploring my neighborhood.

Next thing I know, I just happened to become a fit young woman through pure boredom. These things don't last as we all have discovered in life. I got busy, older, and I gained weight. For the majority of my adult life, I only knew a few exercise tips from that old exercise tape, tried a few fade diets on occasion but mostly relied on hiking and snowboarding to lose those excess pounds.

I even remember college friends that went to the gym regularly were an oddity to me. They'd ask me to join them at times, but I had no idea what I was doing, and it was really boring just trying those pre-made gym circuits. I must have joined a gym about a dozen times before realizing I should stop wasting my money.

Eventually, those hikes and snowboarding adventures became my only go-to to stay fit. This set the stage for my fitness and mindset for much of my life. Now enter my thirties. Finding time to hike every day or the money to have a ski pass every season started to diminish while my waistline slowly increased. Not to mention I started working in the restaurant industry as a side gig and there was a lot of great food, wine and bread to be eaten for free.

I simply couldn't say no to free food, even if I wasn't hungry. I remember looking in the mirror and believing that I simply didn't have the genetics to look fit and lean. My arms would always look like tree trunks and I'd never have abs. My body would just remain shapeless. So was my lot in life. That still didn't make me happy or satisfied with my body and, one day, I had some friends who did the entire three months of the P90X program and got pretty good results.

I figured I'd give it a try! First things first, I started a fade diet. I did the Adkins program for a few months and lost a few pounds. Now I'm feeling pretty good! Then, I committed to the P90X program. I got some results from my efforts but not the same as my friends, but I also didn't watch my diet during that time. With just a little extra muscle and the satisfaction that I could at least commit to three months of working out, I wanted to keep going.

Next, I bought the Insanity program and fizzled out in the first week. It was very intense, and I was losing steam fast by now. I wasn't finding anything that was sustainable. My workouts slowly diminished all together and I ate what I wanted again. Anything that I lost, I gained back again. How frustrating! Back to square one. A big part of me didn't want to slide backward too far regardless of my lack of proper diet and exercise.

I tried to join a running club, meeting once a week to do a 5K. I was so deconditioned that I started with walking most of these runs and gradually got to running more and more. I went to yoga in the parks, I joined a kickball team. Of course, I ended these active days with many beers and more bar food, figuring I deserved it after all that hard work. I was single at this time, which made hiking alone super boring and slightly depressing.

I'm social and enjoy these experiences with others. This was just another excuse not to be as active as I had been in the past. The old mindset that this is how my body would always look slowly crept back in. Even when I did get slightly fit, I knew how dedicated I had to be to get there. That can be a little daunting to do all over again when you slide backward. It takes a while for my body to start to adapt and show change and this was also very demotivating.

I continued to do a quick purge of all "evil" carbs whenever there was a life event that I wanted to look my best for. Yes, it worked for the moment, but by the time I arrived at such event, I ate and drank all I wanted. It was my reward for all my hard work. Coming home, I felt exhausted and working out was not in the cards. At this point, I lived in Alaska where the winters are dark, cold, and depressing.

I had the great idea to join the most expensive gym because it was pretty, cheerful and, most importantly, bright. The spa area was a great perk as well. I took a tour and joined immediately. I had to work another job to pay for this membership too. Thinking that would continue to motivate me, I was wrong yet again.

With no knowledge of what I should be doing when I was even there, I soon got bored again and mostly went to this luxury gym to enjoy the sauna. I was at a loss for what to do next. Despite my failed attempts to get any kind of definition in my body, I knew that out of those times I tried fade diets and my brief stint of working out every day for a few months was: I proved to myself that I can commit to something that has a lot of structure.

That was the biggest mental hurdle to first overcome - commitment. Ok, I got it. Now what? Then, the unexpected happened and I met Michael Parker, the founder of Forge. My mental state was in the right place at that time and I was ready to learn more about nutrition and fitness. He gave me the structure and knowledge that I could finally apply. He taught me about how calories work, portion control and how to make nutritious food choices.

It's so simple and yet I never really researched or comprehended this before. Once my food and calorie intake became better managed, he taught me the basics of exercise and what your body is doing under resistance training and cardio. He wrote me an easy beginner body weight routine that I did every day at home. I finally got the insight, wisdom, and recommended structure from a professional on how to properly exercise and look at food. Outstanding! I started to see major results in just a month.

I couldn't believe it. Over time, I got lean, strong, and quickly became the most in-shape I had been in for years. This was the turning point for the rest of my life! I just needed that scientific structure to find true, long-lasting success. I went back to the gym but now I knew what to do and how to do it well.

Sadly, this was also the first time in my life that I experienced fit shaming. I had no idea this was a thing. I lost around 15lbs and my body looked quite different. Yet, next thing I know, I had people say how I looked too skinny or unhealthy. That I was obsessed with my food and how bad that was.

Trying to explain that not eating 5 slices of pizza is better for me and is not an obsessive habit was hard. I just had to ignore these people and keep doing what I felt was right for me and made me happy. I wasn't doing this for them, I was doing it for me.

Some of the ways I've continued to keep motivated on my new-found fitness and nutrition journey is to keep it fresh. Not only does your body need change to keep progressing, I needed to feel excited to try a new workout or sport. The tangible progression of lifting heavier with better posture and form, made me realize what I'm doing is actually working.

That just made me want to keep it up! One of the biggest things that stood out in my mind when I first got leaner, was Michael telling me, "That's great, keep going." That last part about "keep going" made me realize that my mental mindset was wrong all these years because whenever I reached my goal, I would just stop. I never made exercise part of my daily routine or thought I could get better if I kept it up. What a novel idea. I also find it motivating to look at my own fit images when I'm feeling a little soft.

Looking back at how my body adapts and responds after working hard versus comparing myself to a curvy Instagram model's body motivates me more to reach my own achievable goals. I will never have big hips and a naturally giant butt, but I can achieve something good for my body type and I like how I look strong and healthy. What I found most interesting about my fitness journey was the amount of weight I lifted when I started compared to now.

I can now lift much more because I've been doing it for a few years and muscles just get better and stronger with time. It was very inspiring when I could finally do a bicep curl with a 20lb weight, even if it wasn't a lot of reps. To think I started with 5lbs! Recently, I compared how hard it was to do a 15-minute HITT workout a few years ago and now I can do the whole thing without modifications and can catch my breath much faster.

Yet, I think the best example of success was how it applied to my love for the outdoors when my boyfriend and I won the lottery to hike to the top of Half Dome in Yosemite National Park. We heard this can take up to 10 to 12 hours to complete. We got up early and started our journey. It was definitely a challenging hike not just for its distance and incline, but the cable climb at the end required more upper body strength than I thought it would. We totally rocked it! By the time we half walked, half ran to the bottom, it took us 7 hours round trip. Record time and we felt great.

I could not have done that without being in shape. In the end, I found that after trying crazy intense exercise programs and diets, I must find something that is sustainable for a lifetime; since this isn't just about a few weeks or months, it's forever.

I needed to eat healthy food that I like to eat and can manage when eating out. Exercise programs that challenge me but are also achievable because if it doesn't challenge you, it doesn't change you! Days that I feel too tired to work out or don't want to do that third set, I know I won't get any better if I don't push myself and just do it. Grab a heavier weight, jump a little higher or stay a little longer.

I want to be healthy and add strength and endurance to make all my fun activities and sports that much easier to perform. I remind myself often that, "Rome wasn't built in a day" and nor will my body. Each step I take brings me closer to my goals. I also created this mantra to help me: "I will succeed, I am successful, I am strong, I am capable, and I am beautiful." Soon enough, I believe these thoughts and when my head is in the right place, my body will follow.

The biggest key to my success was finally gaining understanding on body types, calories, nutritious foods and how to build an effective exercise program. All of that came from the perk of having a seasoned fitness professional guide me. If anyone wants to start their journey to a healthy lifestyle, I highly recommend hiring a professional to help teach and mentor you if you have questions, even if it's just for a little while.

Once I understood what it takes, suddenly taking the steps to be healthier didn't seem so daunting and were attainable. Never give up and go be the best version of yourself today!

HEATHER'S COACHING NOTES

Heather is a great example of someone that has struggled with the phenomenon of repeated fitness failure. Throughout her entire life, she has lost, gained, lost and gained body fat because she could not find the mechanism for lasting change.

This is quite common, and most people get stuck in this trap of trying fad diets, fitness programs and other gimmicks to temporarily solve a long-term problem. For Heather, the real hindrance was her basic habits related to food and a sedentary life outside of snow sports and the occasional hike.

While she certainly enjoys being active and fit, she struggled to find the right combination for herself. Like most people, she has tried just about every mainstream fitness or nutrition fad only to see limited periods of moderate success.

The cycle of joining a gym only to cancel it after a time or jump on some silly diet to lose fat only to gain it back plus some breeds discouragement. Like Heather, most people do not understand the underlying issues are not necessarily fitness and nutrition-related.

Attitude, application of knowledge and habit are the primary forces that act as the root cause. Heather realized that her selective knowledge and inconsistency needed to be addressed so she could perform in her activities. Moreover, she made a significant adjustment to her attitude about food and fitness concepts.

When I met Heather almost seven years ago, she was coming out of another cycle of fitness failure with a keto-based fad diet and unhappy with her physique and performance. She was trying so hard to find a solution and this drove her to try all the popular and well-advertised gimmicks to see truly little return or lasting change.

We began by addressing her food volume and quality compared to her activity. We established appropriate caloric goals to ensure she could perform but also maintain a reasonable deficit to inspire the body to convert stored fat for energy. She is incredibly active, and I suspected her food and lack of structured workouts were a major hindrance.

I created a baseline meal plan approach for her and built periodized workouts designed to deliver relatively predictable results. She had made a significant adjustment to her attitude and internal speech and this gave her the renewed determination to give improving her wellness another go.

Heather's determination and joyful spirit needed to be tied into her wellness management. I knew if she could see some progress in short order, she would be unstoppable; she just needed a spark of success. Heather followed the program recommendations carefully and withing just a few months, had radically transformed her composition and increased her strength.

Yes, Heather did experience fit shaming, and this was a major pain point for her. She was disappointed that her friends reacted poorly to her desire to improve herself. I want to clarify this by saying Heather went from a soft 150lbs to a solid and well-formed 130lbs. She went from a shapeless physique to well defined and lean.

She was not underweight, unhealthy or otherwise acting in a destructive manner. Yet many people in her friend group seemed to have had poor attitudes about fitness. Misery loves company. Because Heather is one of the most social people I have ever met, this really hurt her.

Over time, Heather reconciled this and was able to finally feel happy and contented with her newfound love of fitness. She has learned to ignore jealous comments people can make about her attention to her wellbeing and has accomplished some incredible personal bests.

She never gives up and her determination and desire to push her own physical boundaries have paid off for her over and over. Hiking Half Dome from Curry Village to the top and then back to the village in less than seven hours is quite remarkable. For Heather, fitness is a way of life and allows her to do what she loves and look good doing it. Be like Heather, never give up.

Enjoy this free preview of a chapter from
"The 90-Day Habit Transformation"
by Michael S. Parker

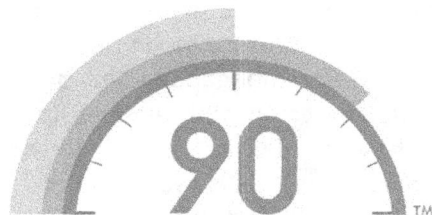

MICHAEL S. PARKER
CPT, NASM, NESTA, FMS

90

DAYHABIT
TRANSFORMATION
HOW TO CREATE
SUSTAINABLE FITNESS AND
NUTRITION SUCCESS

Featuring a *90-Day Habit Workbook* to walk
you through the transformation step-by-step

THE BASICS OF HABIT
"Habit alteration is a slow process and quitting won't speed it up."

I define habits as an acquired set of behaviors that have become almost involuntary, rooted deep in our subconscious through patterns and instigated responses. These learned responses are reinforced by repetition and the more powerful habits are often accompanied by an emotional trigger or instigator.

As an arching theme, habit tendencies are usually linked to the avoidance of pain or pursuing pleasure. Habits result from efficiency adaptations, but for our purposes, we will focus more on the instigators, actions, and rewards toward fitness and nutrition. Generalized habits alone are not good or bad, but the nature of the habit can be classified based on your relationship with the activity.

For example, the habit of brushing one's teeth is positive and the benefits are unquestionable. However, fanatic or obsessive brushing and flossing can cause damage to tooth enamel and gums. The habit of binge eating after a stressful day is certainly not healthy behavior, but a balanced and nutrient-dense food intake is.

We can site hundreds of examples where a regular activity can become an instigator or obsession forming a negative habit. Developing habits and the repetitive execution of behavior or autonomous acts are only the beginning. There must be some sort of reward driving the actions, but they are only the result of an internal or external instigator. In a later chapter, I dive deeply into a concept called the "Power of Conscious Response" but want to make a few notes about habit before we get to that part.

Habits Are Efficiency Adaptations

Habits create continuity, efficiencies, and reward in our daily activities. The automation of response is a necessary component of human function as not every single decision can be made intentionally. Therefore, we must be proactive in our formation of habits, especially those with consequences and prioritize our efforts there.

Diverting energies to effecting personal change based on your projected outcome will be critical for success. Yet, it would be impossible to try and stop every moment in time or interrupt interactions so you can deliberate on a course of action or respond. Our minds want to formulate efficiencies just like our bodies. In exercise physiology, we call this the General Adaptation Syndrome theory tied to periodization.

Essentially, with stress or repetition, the biomechanical and neuromuscular aspects of the human body create efficiency adaptations to accommodate the demand allowing for higher levels of performance. However, adaptation efficiencies in your body are not always positive, just like habit efficiencies are not always positive. To clarify, in exercise physiology, adaptations can serve to positively increase mobility, neuromuscular coordination and strength.

Yet, negative adaptations from a sedentary lifestyle or poor posture cause mobility issues, joint malalignment or decreased performance. In the formation of habit efficiencies, progress would be considered a positive habit, while a regression would be a negative habit. In exercise, you have plateaus, overtraining and undertraining, but the principle of efficiency is the same so that's why I compare them because you must be consciously proactive and apply the proper stresses to elicit the desired result.

As I stated earlier, with positive wellness-based habit formation, we must apply a deliberate set of actions based on a known instigator, a planned response and reward in line with our outcome objective. We can't be a passenger on this ride and must be completely engaged in our conscious response.

Therefore, it is so important we take time to identify those negative or destructive habits that are automated and pay them special attention for alteration. Otherwise, we just get stuck in an automated and destructive response cycle.

Habit and Resistance - Oscillation

We will resist changing or adding a new habit for several reasons. Even though we all know change is inevitable, we resist because it pulls us out of homeostasis, removes predictability and instigates the fear of loss. Let's talk about homeostasis first, as that is one of the more interesting aspects in my estimation because it affects many of our internal systems.

Homeostasis is simply a state of stability physically, mentally and environmentally. The biggest homeostatic conflict I see with my new clients and most people starting a fitness program is oscillation. It is essentially a massive overcorrection, which leads to negative feedback and regression. The most common example is that of the crash or fad dieter.

For a few years now, I have worked with a young lady who used to go through periods of oscillation based on what she saw on social media. While her tendency to suddenly want to uproot her entire training approach and food program have diminished greatly, it is still something she must be conscious of.

When we first met, she was just coming out of a several-month stint with what looked like some kind of Paleo diet having just spent the past three months before that on a restrictive ultra-low-fat diet where she eliminated nearly all fat other than fish. No nuts, no grains, no legumes, no seeds, no oils, no red meats, no poultry, no eggs or avocado. From a dietary standpoint, that is a total opposite in food choice reversal in less than 6 months.

She had an estimated sedentary output of approximately 1,900 calories and was taking in about 800-1,000 and that was about the same consumption on both the super low-fat diet and then the Paleo hybrid. During the time she was on the low-fat diet, she was also doing an extremely aggressive and popular Olympic lift style workout 3-4 days each week, so her probable output was near the 2,300-2,600 mark.

Like most people not properly conditioned for this trendy workout style, she inevitably got injured and decreased her activity. In her convalescence, she followed a social media "influencer" who was a professional exerciser and advertiser all about Paleo and those stupid "booty band" workouts.

You know, the ones where they focus almost exclusively on building the butt and do a half-billion squats and lunges, step-ups and so on with an excessive arch in the low back to make sure its worthy of Instagram to get as much attention as possible. So, she ditched the aggressive workout style and the low-fat diet and went all-in on the booty workouts and Paleo diet.

Anyhow, over the six months, she went from one extreme to another, her composition barely changed at all. The only success she was having was making herself miserable, resenting fitness and inevitably just crashing on her diet. She would gain weight, freak out and overreact to a new fad program. Same formula as every fad, which is caloric restriction, demonization of a macro and overemphasis on a single food source.

I spent several weeks having to build trust with her because she expected to jump into another fad diet and wanted instant results. The problem was we did not have a proper baseline to work with, and her impatience was circumventing the usual application of moderation and consistency in program design and nutritional intake.

I suggested we just hit the reset button and trust the process. She had nothing to lose, and after some gentle mindset coaching, she found balance. I started her with a simple calorically appropriate and nutritionally dense set of menu suggestions, approximately 1,400-1,500 calories, with around 40% from complex carbohydrates, 30% protein and 30% fats.

I also built her a structured fitness program that was periodized so we could validate the results and apply stressors in a systematic way to elicit a predictable outcome. Of course, she melted down at the idea of eating over 1,000 calories and not switching her workouts each week. She had been thoroughly brainwashed by the media and idiotic social media trainers peddling garbage preying on the fears and hopes of the vulnerable.

More than that, she had never built healthy habits based on discipline but rather short-term obsession. We will cover obsession versus discipline in a later chapter, but my point is, she had oscillated so often she had never really formed any constructive habits. What she did was create an unhealthy relationship with food and grew to despise exercise.

On top of all that, she feared change. Her homeostasis was oscillation and by causing her to slow the distance that pendulum swung caused fear. If the program was not extreme, her mind could not reconcile potential effectiveness. She thought nutrition was about starving all day and workouts were supposed to be painful.

On the bright side, the proper application of exercise and responsible energy intake resulted in her finally dropping several percent of body fat in just a few months. Her lean tissue went from 72 lbs to nearly 77 lbs in about four months. She still has tendencies to come to a coaching call questioning nearly every aspect of a new workout plan, but that's also part of her personality.

Habit and Resistance – Selective Knowledge

Very few people enjoy looking foolish or feeling ignorant. It is why we fear public speaking, the first day of school or dating, for example. In fitness, the lack of knowledge ties into the fear of failure we will explore soon, but we will look at how too much or a lack of knowledge can create habit resistance.

I see this in two forms, the first is arrogance or subscription to dogma where people research, compare and digest as much information about their choice as possible. These people are looking to validate their decisions, ensure they have a structure and there are aspects of tribalism present in most cases.

The second resistance is ignorance, confusion from conflicting information or not understanding what approach is best for oneself. These folks do not understand where to start, what to eat, how to exercise or manage their wellbeing. In both cases, we see selective application of knowledge, which in its own way, is a form of resistance.

In the first scenario of the arrogantly educated, many people can get tied up in a specific kind of workout or diet plan and become unwilling to explore alternatives. This is the case even if the subscribed approach is no longer or never has worked, which baffles me. I see this very frequently with diets, but it happens with fitness modalities as well.

Supposed knowledge becomes a resistance when we are comfortable, or our peer group is involved so we don't have to think. Tribalism is often key here, as seen in just about every popular workout style or fad diet. The media also plays a big role, especially with hyper popularized fads. "If this many people are doing it, it must work, right?" Wrong.

But we become emotionally connected to specific approaches and resist change even if what may have been effective for a period, is now producing little or no return. For example, The Keto diet was awesome initially and you lost all this weight, which was cool and that reinforced your subscription to the approach. Then over time, you find this diet is unsustainable for you, so your results and adherence wains.

Where oscillation is not the response, we cling to many aspects of what worked in the past. I have been working with a young woman for many years and when we first met, she was a Keto disciple. Her results had waivered significantly, and with her schedule, she could not maintain the preparation and focus to remain in ketosis. But she was ultra-resistant to any other food lifestyle and over the first few months, she kept trying to incorporate Keto although it was not reasonable.

On top of this, she had a specific vegetarian diet as well. No gluten, no grains, no meats of any kind and restrictive. Her intake rarely exceeded 1,000 calories and she was a restaurant server by day, barkeeping by night and exercised four to five times each week. Her average output was nearly 2,300-2,600 calories each day. Her workouts were not very intense, she was always fatigued, and she resented her fitness and food lifestyle.

It took months of coaching, but finally, she relented and moved to a more balanced and reasonable lifestyle and was able to manage a vegetarian intake. We altered her from five workouts each week to only three with the intention of higher intensity and focus. Her caloric intake was increased to 1,900 with an average deficit of about 250-500 calories, so she experienced less fatigue and all but lost the desire to binge late night. She was doing great for nearly a year and then decided she wanted to try Keto again.

She felt there were inherent health benefits to it based on her previous bias and her ongoing YouTube education. Now that her body composition was where she wanted it, she returned to her failed belief system. Fine. I helped her transition smoothly and within two months, she hit a wall and regressed.

Although Keto was her dogmatic preference, she could not even make it work in her life. She would go through cycles of resistance and regressions. This is a self-imposed problem and being flexible in your approach allows for a higher level of satisfaction and consistency without the cycling failures. She has recently reembraced the reasonable vegan lifestyle she can manage and has abandoned the Keto approach. She is doing great again.

In our second scenario, we have the beginners or the people who have extraordinarily little functional knowledge about fitness or nutrition. The lack of knowledge creates resistance because people fear injury, not seeing results, judgment, disruption to predictable comfort and recognizing they must put forth the effort. Learning something new, especially if you don't want to, can be a powerful resistance.

This group is particularly susceptible to latching onto small pieces of information and forming an unfounded resistance. I have a rare but interesting case example. One of my long-time clients with whom I work with on mindset coaching and advanced fitness likes to supplement our work together with a small group, High-Intensity Interval Training class.

One of her very overweight co-workers who was less than a novice in fitness and nutrition noticed her results and wanted to get involved. My client explained to her how she meets with me every other week on video chat and the level of detail we developed for her fitness programming and nutrition coaching. She also explained she supplements with the live group class twice each week.

However, her co-worker did not want to attend a live class because of her extremely deconditioned state. Yet she selectively heard and held onto the notion of HIIT training and believed it was the right way to work out and anything else was wrong or dangerous. But her medical situation, condition level, joint health, and proprioceptive response were very debilitated.

This situation is grounds to avoid aggressive exercise, jumping and movements like burpees because they are not the correct application of stress. She was well over 280 lbs with acquired diabetes and had never formally exercised in her life.

I explained to her that based on her condition, we would need to start with fundamentals focused on mobility, joint integrity and progressive application of stress to ramp up to HIIT.

Despite my experience and knowledge, she clung to the idea of HIIT because of my other client's success and what she read about HIIT online. She was not actually looking to make a habitual change; she was looking for a quick fix and thought HIIT would be the answer. Over a few sessions, I worked to gain rapport and trust to overcome resistance so I could outline a progressive plan that moved her from the habits that got her to the condition she was in.

I showed her how to understand nutritional basics and incorporate appropriate exercise structure in a prudent manner. I use her as an example because, from the very beginning, she had unusual resistance.

Essentially, I discovered she was trying to find a way to eat candy bars, ice cream, and pizzas without changing habits or exercising consistently. She thought that if she worked out hard a few times, restricted calories or followed macros, she could eat anything she wanted.

Her lack of knowledge became a resistance because she did not seek to learn but instead would find snippets of selective information that supported her poor food choices. Thus, a lack of knowledge can be deliberate. On the bright side, those people who are serious about improving become less resistant to altering their habits.

Results inevitably follow once they open their minds, learn what works for them and eliminate resistance. But it is a decision one must make and commit to. She never did and has since returned to her sedentary and destructive lifestyle.

Habit and Resistance – Return Versus Effort

Of all the habit resistances, return versus effort is the most cynical and surprisingly common. Essentially, this is when we resist making change because we fear the effort will be greater than our perceived return. It is usually tied to the fear of disruption and the fear of exhaustion. When we evaluate our lifestyle and any changes to it, we generally act in pursuing pleasure or the avoidance of pain. Ironically, resistance in this form only delays return even further. You get nothing for nothing.

The comfort of predictability and pain we already know can sabotage the development of healthy habits. We settle for the familiar pain instead of the potential unknown pain of change. Often, people who resist in this manner have experienced repeated failed attempts to alter their habits or wellness. They know how hard it was last time and the results were not commensurate to their effort.

Yet when we examine these cases, we find that the attempt was almost always through a gimmick, fad diet or incorrect exercise approach. Another observation is that people jump on programs with a specified timeline and never actually change root habits to accommodate a lifestyle. Like I said earlier, your efforts must exceed the 90 days of institutional change outlined within this book.

The good news is lack of knowledge and misdirection of energy is a problem we can solve. I have two examples to share with you related to the resistance of return versus effort. First, I have worked with a young lady for quite some time and this resistance is her primary roadblock. She is well organized and has all aspects of her wellness needs aligned. She has meals delivered to her, a gym in her community complex and a gym at work.

She meets with me every single week and has the support of her husband and teenage son. She has her workouts scheduled for five days each week and they are built specifically to her needs. The problem is, she comes to her coaching calls with less than a quarter of her workouts completed nearly every week. Why? Everything is set and all she must do is execute her workouts.

She is resisting because she is afraid that if she does the workouts, she will see no return and it won't be worth it. I recently said to her, "Well, you are getting the exact same outcome you are trying to avoid by not doing the work." That seemed to resonate, and she slowly has been improving with exercise adherence. She has nothing to lose by just doing her workouts. They are only 45 minutes and when she does them, she always reports feeling better.

Granted, she has her nutrition dialed and has significantly improved her mindset and lifestyle in general. Yet she was not achieving her potential because of her avoidance of activity.

The funny thing is, when I wrote this, it has been five weeks of her hitting every workout and she has reduced her body fat by over one percent, which relates to just under three pounds of fat for her. Imagine where she would be now if she did not resist when she started nine months ago.

The second example is on the extreme side and I only encounter this intensity of resistance infrequently, but I feel it's worth examining. I worked with a woman for about three months that resisted everything. I don't think I am exaggerating much when I say "everything" either. She refused to work out, refused to track her food for any period, refused to clean house and manage her environments and refused to consider any self-reflection at all.

Meaning when I had her do the weekly homework in the 90-day workbook, it was incomplete or not done at all. She was very pleasant, and we had nice conversations and rapport, but she simply resisted everything in the politest defiance ever. I really wanted to understand her inability to simply make some small alterations to achieve the very purpose for which she hired me. After one of our last coaching calls, she revealed that because she was so intensely obese and deconditioned, she felt it would be too hard to ever get well, so why bother.

She had crossed over so far that she believed the effort was not worth all the rewards of fitness. She had tried so often over twenty years to correct her life path, but she was so ingrained and comfortable with her pain that the anticipated new and unknown pain of change would be too much. She also tried to buy her fitness.

She enrolled in a major coaching or clinical program every few years and her history was to quit or not adhere. She spent thousands and thousands of dollars and never followed through.

This is because the act of purchasing a program gave her just a moment of gratification and hope, but when it came time for the work, she was not truly ready to change. She had a deep set of limiting beliefs and in the stages of change, she never got past the Preparation phase, which we will review the chapter after next.

Habit and Resistance – Fear

Fear of change can be quite subtle and elusive from your conscious realization on the one hand or be obvious and identifiable on the other. The level of fear and associated resistance varies from person to person, but we all feel it. Fear born anxiety is double-edged because it can inspire action or cause paralysis, so it is important to courageously meet fears head-on and address the source of your resistance and act. Let's address some common fear-based resistances such as disruption of homeostatic routine, fear of failure, fear of guilt and fear of exhaustion.

Fear of Disruption

Disruption of homeostatic routine is simply the fear of having your comfort zone or habits challenged. It's fascinating that even our negative routines that have greatly influenced our discontented state can impede our desire to make a change. We must eliminate the fear of disruption by addressing solutions that will resolve the negative consequences of our behavior. When we are comfortable, we become complacent. Let's look at an example of how to positively disrupt deconstructive habits based on the comfort of routine.

I work with a gentleman who has spent several years in the relative comfort of predictability but had suffered significant health-related issues because of the level of destructive homeostatic comfort. He contacted me to help him make a change and overcome the fear because he was finding the quality of his life was deteriorating in several areas, and his homeostatic routine was a major factor. He is a traveling salesperson on the road about every other week or so and the nature of his profession requires a good deal of sitting in meetings, dining with clients and long hours.

In his spare time, he would play online video games or binge-watch television shows compounding the negative effects of a low activity level profession, with a sedentary personal lifestyle. The fear of changing his routine was double-pronged because he could not see a solution to meetings or long hours. He also contributed much of his professional success to his dinner and cocktail meetings and was afraid to change his sales and client retention approach because he felt these interactions were a primary reason for his rapport and later success with clients.

On the other prong, he found levity and escape from the rigors of his job by playing video games with a group of other gamers. His television shows also allowed him to disconnect. In our coaching sessions, we created a more inclusive mindset related to his work, hobbies, and wellness. I like to work backward by identifying how aspects of one's life improve with higher levels of fitness, nutrition management and overall sense of wellbeing.

We often attempt to compartmentalize fitness in one box, nutrition in another, and then further separate work from personal life. This is an unrealistic approach, and we must strive to make our lives more inclusive, which I will explore in the later chapter. Once we agree that all aspects of our lives cannot effectively be rigidly compartmentalized or quarantined, we can work to create positive inclusivity based on flexible or rigid boundaries.

In my example case, we had to ratify why his fitness and food choices were important and how to make this inclusive. We came up with several strategies for his client meals and cocktail hours by improving food choice, serving size and volume of drinking.

This allowed him to make better choices within the conditions of his work life, which ultimately translated to his personal life.

As a side note, when he and his partner would go to dinner, he automatically made better choices without sacrificing the value of dinning out and sharing time with his significant other. He overcame his fear of damaging his career by simply changing his self-imposed rules to be in line with his wellness goals. He did not need to sacrifice his professional approach, but his initial fear did not allow him to consider any alternatives or see the solution was quite simple.

Now, we had to address his sedentary personal lifestyle and the poor food choices made from convenience. This was more difficult because he did not want to eliminate his time spent with video games. No problem. We agreed that he would do a 30-minute workout prior to gaming, and instead of ordering pizza, which was his routine, he would have a nutritious meal prepared. We eliminated the negative consequences of making a poor food choice of convenience by having a healthy alternative.

He did not have to sacrifice gaming, and he made a once a week allowance for sharing a small pizza with his partner provided, he did a full hour workout beforehand. The half pizza was also contingent on a commitment he did at least four of his scheduled five workouts that week despite how busy things got. He also limited his television viewing significantly and used that time to exercise instead. By applying inclusive principles, setting boundaries and making minor alterations to his choices, he maintained the areas of his life he most valued.

He still wines and dines clients and prospects, plays video games, eats pizza occasionally and has developed healthy personal boundaries. He has gone from a completely sedentary life void of exercise to exercising consistently well over five days each week. He has fundamentally transformed his attitude toward fitness and nutrition and incorporates wellness into his general mindset. He has turned his negative homeostatic routine into a positive homeostatic routine, which provides that comfort of predictability without the damage.

Fear of Failure

Fear is a paralyzing agent in fitness and nutrition lifestyle management for several reasons. First, we fear we are choosing the wrong fitness activity or diet plans. We become so inundated with contradictory information that we fear choosing the wrong path and wasting time, money, motivation and not seeing progress. Second, procrastination is a common problem we must overcome to maintain our focused workouts and discipline around food choices.

The procrastination just reinforces the fears and we justify why we can't seem to make it work. It's quite a vicious cycle and can be hard to break unless you are applying the Power of Conscious Response and setting reasonable goals for yourself. Another paralyzer is the fear of not being fit enough to start a workout plan or go to the gym in general. We fear we may be judged or look foolish, trying to figure out a machine and perhaps perform exercises incorrectly.

Many people fear over-soreness or exacerbating an old injury so it's easy to avoid even starting. I have even heard people say they want to wait to hire a trainer until after they get back in shape. This makes no sense at all and is just another form of fear manifesting procrastination. My experience has shown me the excuse of not hiring a professional until you are in better shape is usually the fear of wasting money.

We doom our wellness journey from the beginning because we have experienced so much fitness failure in the past, it is now our expected outcome.

I will cover fitness failure later, but suffice to say, it is the common outcome for most Americans. I am sure some people may feel embarrassed about their condition and suspect a trainer would be judgmental, so they avoid it. I have seen foolish trainers use belittlement or other divisive approaches thinking they are motivating, but this is a terrible coaching technique. Sadly, some celebrity trainers made themselves famous and built whole brands on yelling at clients, which has been popular on national reality television. This is an appalling practice and is a false representation of most fitness professionals.

Finally, fear can be completely counterintuitive and when tied to extremes, produce a strong resistance. Dozens of clients have attached to an approach and have a very hard time detaching even though it is clearly not working. They fear the change will make things worse and so doggedly cling to the mast of a sinking ship. Don't be afraid to fail because it's not about whether you fail, it's about whether you keep trying.

One of the most common I experience is in young women. Imagine a woman who is between 5' 10" and 6' who at one point ate 800-1,000 calories each day as a teenager and young adult while exercising several times each week but not necessarily in a structured manner. The grace of youth forgives many mistakes, but as she ages, her metabolic and hormonal responses can change significantly.

Now this woman is in her early 30s and noticing a decrease in her performance and her body composition. She becomes soft and her figure becomes less defined and finds herself getting ill or injured often. Let's say her exercise output has changed to a very structured and demanding system of progressive workouts and her estimated caloric output is between 2,500-3,000 calories each day.

Yet she refuses to move from an 800-calorie intake because of fear. Clearly, her output demands energy but absent calories provided by food intake, how will the body make up this deficit? It will affect the internal structures and convert energy there. Muscle mass is converted, glycogen stores are low, and the sympathetic nervous system is activated and likely the cause for a compromised immune system.

I lost track of how often I have worked with someone stuck in this trap. They get their workouts dialed and execute flawlessly each week only to not see results. Their own fear is causing this and if they just trust the obvious, they nearly always see improvement in a matter of days. But getting a young woman off the 800 calories to a more reasonable 2,000 is a coaching challenge.

Effectively, I am asking these ladies to nearly double their habitual intake, and this takes time to overcome. I can say that in my experience over the years, every woman that slowly increased her intake with nutrient-dense foods saw fantastic results because their fitness was already dialed. Once the nutrition comes into play, the results come as well. But it is very scary for these people who have imposed this rigid idea that fewer calories equal better results. They don't.

Fear of Guilt

By my observation, the fear of guilt seems to manifest in two specific forms. On the one hand, some feel guilty before they even start and saturate their thoughts with self-doubt, questioning their decisions and feeling generally dissatisfied. On the other hand, I have seen some people allow guilt to drive an obsessive like adherence to certain aspects of a program.

This is especially true with extreme calorie and food journaling. In both cases, guilt drives a strong feeling of responsibility for outcome, and shame gets tied into the feelings of guilt even if there is not a perceivable failure.

As a foundational principle, I suggest caloric counting and exercise adherence be a well-constructed, yet flexible guide based on discipline, not obsession.

Having stated that, I commonly see the first group where doubt and indecisiveness cause paralysis, and that results in feeling guilty, because of the indecisiveness and lack of execution. The guilt is usually because the person feels like they are on the wrong path or their problems are so big that they can't seem to solve them no matter how hard they try. Guilt comes in the form of missing workouts or slipping up on food.

It is common for someone to overeat at lunch and then just throw the rest of the day away and binge because they felt they already failed. Guilt is especially strong where someone is suffering from an eating disorder and can't seem to defeat it. The feelings of being so completely controlled by something like anorexia, bulimia, obsessive macro and calorie counting, or other disorders that cause many to stay stuck in the cycle.

Look at bulimia, for example. Guilt fuels a binge, guilt fuels a purge, guilt fuels self-loathing, then guilt triggers binging, and it repeats. I have worked with dozens of women and men stuck in a cycle, and they are hesitant to start any program because they fear if they pay attention to it, they will obsess on it and the cycle will activate. Sadly, many of their needs exceed my scope of practice, so I refer them to a clinician, but I still support the basics of a designed exercise plan for these clients in conjunction with a mental health caregiver if they choose to do so.

It's heartbreaking how many stories I could share around this topic, and if you experience these feelings or are suffering from an eating disorder, know there is hope, and you can get out of the cycle.

It is hard, and you may have relapse and feelings of defeat, but I have seen so many people pull themselves out of this destructive situation. You can do it, so never give in.

One of my favorite clients suffers aggressively from bulimia with intense feelings of guilt, fear, and shame. She has struggled from the time she was a teenager and is now in her early 30s but still fighting. Some of our coaching calls are just letting her cry and work through her thoughts. She has several awesome weeks, and suddenly, she will message me letting me know she spent the last two days binging and purging to the point of exhaustion.

I must modify her workouts often to accommodate and help support her needs as best I can. Her clinician has had her stop food journaling for reasons related to obsessive-compulsive disorder, and we reduced her workouts to low impact just to keep the habit of working out. Plus, she always feels better after exercise, and we have found that strength training is one of her new favorites, and she is less likely to skip.

She particularly loves circuit training because we can do it in a half-hour and she need not think, she can just do. She is working on overcoming this intense guilt and finding her internal strength. A special note to her: You light the lives of others and your value is immeasurable. Your quality is not dictated by the past and the pain there, it is in the future you are making. Find your joy.

Fear of Exhaustion

And here we come to my personal fear-based habit resistance, and I suspect it is shared by millions of hard-working people. For me, it's not so much about the habit of exercise, but more in knowing I have been working twelve or more hours and still need to complete my workout.

I must be very sharp for my client calls, writing, research, and programming, and it is easy to resist the structure of planned workouts and justify based on time and exhaustion.

I already have a tendency towards insomnia, so that compounds the fear of feeling drained. I see this in almost all my clients to some degree and there are several strategies to overcome this fear. Remember that we can tie excuses such as not having enough time to this as well, but in the end, it's about avoiding the feeling of depletion. This is a simple fear to overcome, but it is not easy. Time management, prioritization and shifting one's mind to make wellness an inclusive part of their lives is quite challenging in practice. However, I have never met anyone who can truly justify a lack of time as a reason to not work out.

There are 168 hours in a week, and you most certainly can find thirty minutes to an hour every other day in there. Let's say you committed to five, 30-minute workouts each week, you still have 165.5 hours left. Even if you slept for only six hours each night, you still have 123.5 hours. Of course, you are an extremely hard worker and put in long hours professionally with an average workday of twelve hours over six of the seven days in the week, leaving 51.5 hours. You are very committed to friends and family, so each day you spend at least five hours with loved ones ringing in 35 hours. This leaves you 16.5 hours weekly, which is 2 extra hours each day.

So why is it you can't seem to fit in exercise? Well, it's not about time, it's about exhaustion. We confuse the two and that is why it is a common fear for folks with busy lives. Occasionally the fear of exhaustion is tied to laziness and lack of prioritization. But laziness is often the result of comparing the perceived return over effort, which creates its own set of resistances.

This concludes the bonus chapter from the
"90-Day Habit Transformation"
By Michael S. Parker

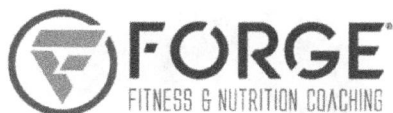
FORGE
FITNESS & NUTRITION COACHING

For more information about Forge Fitness and Nutrition
programming or to enjoy some of Michael's other publications
check out www.forgept.com